Brain Health

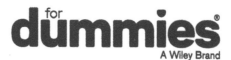

Brain Health

by Sarah McKay, DPhil

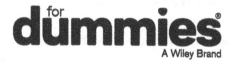

Brain Health For Dummies®

Published by: **John Wiley & Sons, Inc.**, 111 River Street, Hoboken, NJ 07030-5774, www.wiley.com

For general information on our other products and services, please contact our Customer Care Department within the U.S. at 877-762-2974, outside the U.S. at 317-572-3993, or fax 317-572-4002. For technical support, please visit https://hub.wiley.com/community/support/dummies.

Wiley publishes in a variety of print and electronic formats and by print-on-demand. Some material included with standard print versions of this book may not be included in e-books or in print-on-demand. If this book refers to media that is not included in the version you purchased, you may download this material at http://booksupport.wiley.com. For more information about Wiley products, visit www.wiley.com.

Library of Congress Control Number: 2024950290

ISBN 978-1-394-27337-9 (pbk); ISBN 978-1-394-27339-3 (ebk); ISBN 978-1-394-27338-6 (ebk)

SKY10091017_111524

Contents at a Glance

Table of Contents

PART 5: AVOIDING BRAIN HEALTH HAZARDS 275

CHAPTER 17: **Buffering Against Toxic Stress** 277

CHAPTER 18: **Rethinking Drugs and Alcohol** 299

Introduction

Welcome to *Brain Health For Dummies*, your guide to understanding and maintaining a healthy brain throughout your life.

I'm a neuroscientist, which means I spent years in neurobiology research labs exploring the mysteries of the mind, unraveling the complexities of neurons, synapses, and brain networks, and figuring out how our thoughts, emotions, and behaviors come together and what happens when they're damaged.

These days, I focus on translating the latest neuroscience research into practical, brain health tips anyone can use. Or, as I like to say, I explain the brain!

As you read this book, think of me as a part neuroscientist, part tour-guide, here to help you navigate and appreciate what I believe is the coolest thing in the universe: your brain!

Maybe you hope to boost your memory, manage stress better, or understand how your lifestyle choices affect your brain. Perhaps you're deeply concerned about a loved one's mental health, or you're caring for someone with dementia and want to avoid the same fate. Or maybe you're a parent looking to give your kids the best start in life by understanding how to nurture their developing brains. Whatever your goals, age, or life stage, this book will guide you in understanding and maintaining a healthy brain.

About This Book

This book gives you a practical guide to understanding your brain and keeping it in tip-top shape. It's not just about avoiding issues like mental health problems or dementia; it's about thriving, feeling great, and being your best self at any age. I've structured the chapters into several parts, each addressing different aspects of brain health. Here's a sneak peek:

>> **Introduction to Brain Health:** Learn about the brain's structure and function. You'll look at the tools, tests, and gadgets used to monitor brain

health, dig into disorders like ADHD and Alzheimer's Disease, and explore quirky brain traits. Plus, I'll break down the numbers on risk factors, genetics, and lifestyle choices, making it all easy to understand.

>> **Charting Brain Health at Different Ages and Stages:** Here, you'll examine how brain health evolves from childhood through adolescence to old age. I'll discuss critical periods of brain development, the importance of nurturing healthy brains in children, and the challenges of aging gracefully.

>> **Beyond Aging: Other Factors That Impact Brain Health:** This part covers the interplay of sex and gender in brain health, the impact of environmental and technological factors, and the unique challenges faced after brain injuries.

>> **Keeping Your Brain Healthy:** Practical strategies for maintaining and enhancing brain health are covered here. I'll look at the effects of nutrition, exercise, sleep, social engagement, and cognitive challenges on brain health.

>> **Avoiding Brain Health Hazards:** Finally, you'll learn how to buffer against toxic stress, rethink the use of drugs and alcohol, avoid metabolic diseases, and take charge of hearing loss.

Implementing the strategies in this book can boost your brain health, but some conditions need specialized care. If you're even slightly worried, seek professional help. This book is a great resource, but it can't replace personalized care. Start by talking to your family doctor or therapist about how this information can support your treatment. Remember, maintaining brain health is a life-long journey; seeking help is a strength, not a weakness.

Foolish Assumptions

I know brain science can seem intimidating. After all, I've spent my career watching the wide-eyed look people give me at dinner parties when I say what I do. (And no, I can't read your mind!) But don't worry, you don't need to be a doctor, scientist, or even a "rocket surgeon" to get the hang of it. That's because in writing this book, I made a few "foolish assumptions."

First, I figured that you, like many others, are curious about your brain and eager to learn how to take care of it, even if the topic sometimes feels a bit overwhelming. But you're probably not a complete newbie when it comes to taking an interest in health and wellbeing.

Second, I also guessed that you might not have much time on your hands. (Who does these days?) So I've made sure the information is clear and easy to digest.

I also guessed you're not just another person looking for generic advice like "Drink plenty of water" or "Exercise regularly." Whether you're a busy professional juggling a million things, a student cramming for exams, a parent trying to give your kids the best start, a woman navigating midlife brain health challenges, a retiree looking to stay mentally agile, or someone managing a pre-existing condition, I've included something here for everyone.

Icons Used in This Book

Throughout this book, I use icons to highlight different types of information:

Practical advice or helpful insights.

Key points or important information to keep in mind.

More detailed scientific information that you can skip if you're not interested.

Cautionary notes about potential risks to be aware of, or suggestions to seek professional medical advice.

Beyond the Book

In addition to the content within these pages, you can find additional resources online. Visit www.dummies.com and search for "Brain Health For Dummies Cheat Sheet" for extra tips and information.

Where to Go from Here

This book is designed so that you can jump into any chapter that interests you. You don't need to read it from cover — cover although you're welcome to do so! If you're new to the topic, you might want to start with Part 1, where I cover the basics of the brain and brain health. If you're interested in specific topics like childhood, adolescence, women's health or hearing loss, diet, or exercise, feel free to skip ahead to those chapters. Each chapter stands on its own, allowing you to explore the content in any order you like.

Let's start the next chapter in your brain health journey!

1
An Introduction to Brain Health

Explore brain health and discover how to thrive and perform at your best.

Understand your brain by learning about structure and how your nervous system influences how you think, feel, and behave.

Discover how scientists study brain health using advanced research and brain scans.

Learn about brain disorders ranging from neurodevelopmental to mental health conditions.

Calculate your brain health risks by understanding the impact of genetics and lifestyle.

Chapter **1**

Embracing Brain Health Fundamentals

H aving a healthy brain is about more than avoiding mental health problems, diseases, or dementia; it's about thriving, feeling good, and performing at your best.

Some people think being healthy means not being sick, but the World Health Organization sees it differently. They say health is all about "a state of complete physical, mental, and social well-being and not merely the absence of disease or infirmity." This definition also means that health isn't just about eating veggies or keeping cholesterol in check. It's a more holistic view, nicely aligned with what we often call "well-being."

Let's be real: Some brain health conditions are out of our control, thanks to genetics or just plain bad luck. But don't worry! You can do plenty of things to lower your risk or improve symptoms for many diagnoses, diseases, and quirks. Remember, being healthy isn't just about dodging illness; it's about making the most of your brain health, no matter your diagnosis.

Getting to Grips with the Biopsychosocial Model of Health

To truly understand brain health, you need to consider the bio-psycho-social model, which looks at the interplay between biological, psychological, and social factors.

This is not as boring as it sounds!

Taking a bio-psycho-social approach acknowledges that your health is influenced not only by your biology (such as genes, hormones, muscle strength, or gut health) but also by your psychological state (such as your stress levels and mental health) and your social environment (including relationships and community).

I like to put the brain in the middle of the bio-psycho-social model and call it the "Bottom-Up Outside-In Top-Down" model of the brain, shown in Figure 1-1.

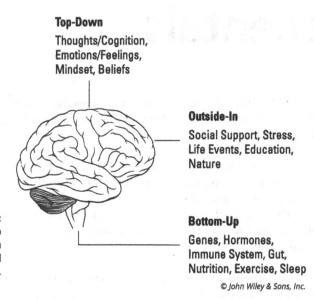

Top-Down
Thoughts/Cognition,
Emotions/Feelings,
Mindset, Beliefs

Outside-In
Social Support, Stress,
Life Events, Education,
Nature

Bottom-Up
Genes, Hormones,
Immune System, Gut,
Nutrition, Exercise, Sleep

© John Wiley & Sons, Inc.

FIGURE 1-1:
The Bottom-Up
Outside-In
Top-Down model
of the brain.

>> **Bottom-Up** elements are the biological or physiological determinants of brain health, development, and aging. The elements include genes, hormones, the immune system, nutrition, exercise, sleep, and the constant streams of data about what's happening inside your body, some of which you're conscious of (such as a full bladder, sore back, or kicking baby), other factors you're unaware of (such as hormone levels or gut pH).

>> **Outside-In** elements are outside in the environment and make their way in via our senses (what you see, hear, smell, touch, and taste). Outside includes your social circle, the culture you grew up in, the built and natural environment, current circumstances, and external stressors.

>> **Top-Down** elements include what you think of as your mind — your conscious thoughts, emotions, personality, language, expectations, and belief systems.

My version of the bio-psycho-social model may help you understand the complex and dynamic nature of brain health. And I remind you of it plenty of times in this book!

Understanding How a Healthy Brain Works

To maintain a healthy brain, it's helpful to understand its main duties.

Your brain is responsible for perceiving the world, interpreting biological signals, guiding behavior, feeling emotions, thinking and reasoning, socializing with others, controlling movement, storing and retrieving memories, and maintaining homeostasis.

Here are a few ways a healthy brain performs when it's in peak condition:

Perceiving your world

Your brain constantly processes sensory information from your environment. This includes everything you see, hear, taste, touch, and smell. The brain's ability to perceive and interpret sensory data enables you to navigate and understand the world. This sensory processing is vital for learning, memory, and everyday functioning.

Interpreting biological signals

Your brain receives and interprets signals from within your body, such as hunger, thirst, and pain. These internal signals are crucial for maintaining homeostasis and responding to your body's needs. Understanding these signals helps you manage your health and well-being more effectively.

Guiding your behavior

Your brain is the command center that guides your actions and decisions. It integrates information, plans, and executes behaviors to help you achieve your goals. Whether performing daily tasks, solving problems, or pursuing long-term objectives, your brain's executive functions are at work.

Feeling emotional

Emotions are an integral part of your brain's function. They influence your thoughts, behaviors, and interactions with others. Emotional health is about recognizing, understanding, and managing your feelings. A well-regulated emotional brain contributes to resilience, mental health, and overall well-being.

Thinking and reasoning

Cognitive functions such as thinking, reasoning, and problem-solving are essential for navigating life's challenges. Your brain's ability to process information, make decisions, and learn new skills is fundamental to personal and professional growth. Cognitive health ensures you can think clearly, remember information, and stay mentally agile.

Socializing and interacting with others

Humans are inherently social beings; our brains are wired for social interaction. Effective communication, empathy, and relationship-building are all functions of a healthy brain. Social connections provide emotional support, reduce stress, and enhance cognitive function. Maintaining a social network (IRL, not online!) is crucial for brain health.

Practical Tips to Get Started

Here are a few practical tips to start improving your brain health right away:

>> **Connect:** Being loved by and connected to others protects against cognitive decline and poor mental health. Socializing is a cognitive workout, involving thinking, feeling, sensing, reasoning, and intuition. Social isolation is as bad for you as smoking, so make sure you stay connected! For more on this topic, check out Chapter 15.

>> **Sleep:** Our biological rhythms are set by the sun. Skimping on sleep affects cognition, mood, and learning and increases the risk of depression and dementia. Healthy sleep consolidates memory, sparks creativity, and smooths emotional edges. Prioritize your sleep for better control over your thoughts and feelings. For lots more on sleep, see Chapter 14.

>> **Nourish:** The secret to longevity isn't in the fine details of diet but in avoiding processed foods. Eat less than you think you need — your brain works best when you're slightly hungry and looking for food. For more on nutrition, see Chapter 12.

>> **Move:** Your brain evolved for movement. Moving your body through the natural world by whatever means you enjoy most is the best exercise for your brain. So, get up and get going! (And read Chapter 13 for more tips on exercising.)

>> **Calm:** Not all stress is bad, but chronic or toxic stress, especially life events that are out of your control, can mess up your mind and brain health. I cover this topic in Chapter 17. The key to handling stress is improving your perceived ability to cope. Find peace in the chaos. Pay attention to your breath, which is a core component of many mindfulness practices — it reduces anxiety and depression and improves sleep.

>> **Nature:** The world around you profoundly impacts your brain and behavior, as I discuss in Chapter 11. You probably already know how refreshing nature can be. You're happier and healthier when surrounded by nature, parkland, or even indoor plants. So, get a bit wild and enjoy the greenery.

>> **Challenge:** Kids love to run and play, while adults tend to take life more seriously. We don't stop playing and learning because we get old; we get old because we stop playing and learning. Staying mentally engaged and challenging yourself reduces the risk of age-related cognitive decline and dementia. There's more on this topic in Chapter 16.

>> **Feel:** "We don't laugh because we're happy; we're happy because we laugh." Embrace the good that comes your way and spiral into positivity. Practicing and repeating positive experiences and emotions leads to better mental and physical health. So, laugh more and savor those moments!

>> **Seek:** Purpose and meaningful work bring positive emotions such as love, compassion, and gratitude, which counteract stress. Living a meaningful life may seem like a strange addition to a neuroscience-based list, but having a purpose correlates with robust brain health, mental health, and even longevity.

>> **Protect:** Hearing loss is more than an inconvenience; it can lead to social isolation depression and increase your risk of dementia. Don't ignore it — check your hearing and use hearing aids if needed. See Chapter 20 for

more advice. And protect your brain from injuries, as I cover in Chapter 10. Wear helmets during risky activities and take steps to prevent falls. Show the youngsters you're still nimble but do it safely!

Your Brain Health Journey Starts Here

This book is designed to be your companion on your brain health journey. Each chapter is packed with information and tips to help you understand and enhance your brain's health.

You embark on a mesmerizing trip, zooming in to explore the microscopic world of neurons, neurotransmitters, and synapses. You zoom out to observe the bigger picture, examine brain scans, study population-wide trends, meet some of the researchers, and read about their work.

It may feel dizzying as you switch perspectives, but don't worry — I'm here to provide a steady hand and guide you through every twist and turn of this incredible neuro-adventure!

IN THIS CHAPTER

» Exploring the brain's architecture and neural pathways

» Investigating neuron connections and synapse functions

» Understanding chemical communication within the brain

» Examining the brain's capacity to adapt and change

» Integrating how the brain's systems work in unison

Chapter **2**

Getting to Know Your Brain and Nervous System

Welcome to the human brain! The place inside your head is more intricate and mysterious than even the most complex constellations strewn across the universe. And if you reach up and pat yourself on the head, just there beneath your fingertips lies the seat of all your thoughts, feelings, a lifetime of memories and dreams. It might seem scary to start this journey of understanding because, let's face it, neuroscience sounds as complex as rocket surgery! But don't worry — getting a sense of the basic structure of your brain and nervous system is the first step to keeping it healthy, and the journey starts in the most familiar place: your own head.

By the end of this chapter, you'll have a basic understanding of how these parts work together to give you a complete picture of neural function that is beautiful and useful for maintaining the health of every brain (yours and those you love).

Navigating Nervous System Anatomy

When you think about brain health, you probably picture the brain alone. However, the nervous system is a network that includes the brain, the spinal cord, and numerous branching nerves reaching out to every organ and muscle, fingertip, and toe in your body.

Mapping the divisions of the nervous system

Neuroscientists typically divide the nervous system into two main divisions and multiple sub-divisions, which you can see in Figure 2-1.

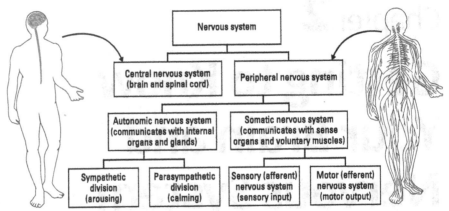

FIGURE 2-1: Divisions of the nervous system.

© John Wiley & Sons, Inc.

The *central nervous system* (CNS) is the body's command center, consisting of the brain and spinal cord. The *brain* is the central integrator for sensory data from both the world around you and your body, directing behavior, cognitive processes, memory encoding, and the body's homeostatic regulation. The *spinal cord*, encased within the spine's vertebrae, is a superhighway for nerve signals between the brain and body, handling swift, reflexive responses.

The *peripheral nervous system* (PNS), which branches out from the CNS, is a vast network of nerves that carries signals to and from the body's organs, muscles, and sensory receptors.

The PNS is divided into the *somatic nervous system,* overseeing voluntary movements, and the *autonomic nervous system,* controlling involuntary functions such as heartbeat and digestion. The latter is split again into the *sympathetic* and *parasympathetic systems,* which work together to gear the body up for action and promote relaxation. Also, part of this intricate network is the *enteric nervous system,* managing the gut independently yet in constant dialogue with the brain, a fascinating topic explored further in Chapter 12.

Digging into the brain's structure and organization

The brain's cortex is indeed deeply folded into ridges (gyri) and grooves (sulci). The folds mean more neurons can be packed into the limited space inside your skull (much like scrunching up tissue paper to stuff into a box).

Mapping the brain's cortex

If you take a bird's eye view of the brain, you'll see it is made of two hemispheres (the left and right hemispheres). Traditionally, the cortex is subdivided into four lobes per hemisphere: frontal, temporal, parietal, and occipital (see Figure 2-2).

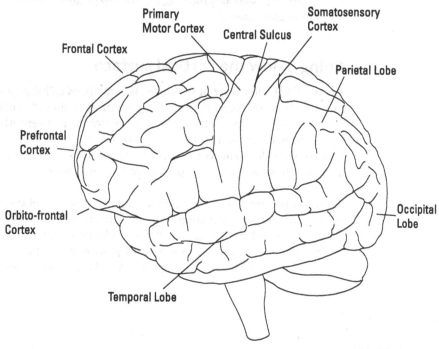

FIGURE 2-2: Lobes of the neocortex.

© John Wiley & Sons, Inc.

This convoluted walnut-like appearance varies from person to person but follows a general pattern that neuroanatomists have meticulously mapped. Each lobe has a few specific jobs that are listed here:

>> **Frontal lobes,** positioned right behind your forehead, are the command center for personality and our ability to communicate and make decisions. The pre-frontal cortex (PFC), located at the very front, is critical for complex cognitive tasks and orchestrating social behavior.

>> **Temporal lobes,** found beneath your temples, act as the brain's auditory processors, allowing you to interpret sounds and language. Deep under the surface of the lobes, the hippocampus plays a crucial role in forming memories and processing emotions.

>> **Parietal Lobes,** situated between the crown of your head and the tips of your ears, are the meeting place for sensory information, weaving together input from touch, taste, and smell, and are essential for understanding spatial orientation and navigation.

>> **Occipital lobes,** located at the very back of your head just above the nape of your neck, serve as the brain's visual processing center, translating signals from your eyes into the images you see.

>> **Cerebellum,** tucked under the occipital lobes at the base of your skull, coordinates voluntary motions, maintaining posture and balance and modulating reflexes.

Going below the cortical surface

The wrinkled outer layer of the cortex is sometimes called *grey matter*, which gets its name from its color! Grey matter comprises brain cells such as neurons and glia (more about both shortly). The *white matter* sits just beneath the cortex, about one centimeter down, as shown in Figure 2-3. It's called white matter because it appears white due to nerve fibers covered in a fatty substance called myelin, which insulates these fibers like the plastic coating on a cable.

White matter tracts serve as communication pathways between the cortical grey matter and deeper processing hubs or clusters of brain cells called *subcortical nuclei*, shown in Figure 2-4. Subcortical nuclei have various jobs including motor control, emotions, memory, and reward processing. Their interactions with the cortex are essential for complex behaviors and cognitive processes.

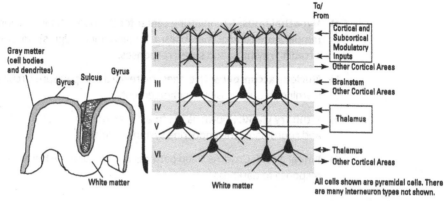

FIGURE 2-3:
Grey matter and white matter.

© *John Wiley & Sons, Inc.*

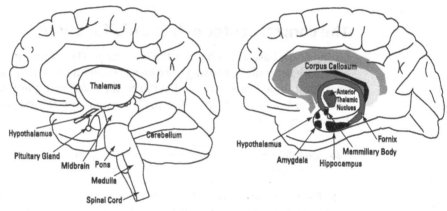

FIGURE 2-4:
Subcortical nuclei and brainstem.

© *John Wiley & Sons, Inc.*

Some of the more important subcortical nuclei and their main roles include:

>> **Thalamus:** The brain's grand central station for sensory information (excluding smell), channeling signals from the senses to the cortex for processing.

>> **Basal ganglia:** Responsible for coordinating movement, storing automatic movements and habits, influencing decision-making, and emotional cognition.

>> **Amygdala:** Central to processing emotions, it tags experiences with emotional significance, and is essential for storing emotional memories.

>> **Hippocampus:** Plays a key role in forming memories and spatial navigation. It holds short-term memories and transfers them for long-term storage, often during sleep.

- >> **Hypothalamus:** A monitoring center for the body's vital functions, including temperature control, metabolism, hunger, thirst, aggression, sexual arousal, circadian rhythms, and stress responses.

- >> **Nucleus accumbens:** Oversees the reward and pleasure circuits, facilitating learning through positive reinforcement.

- >> **Pituitary gland:** Known as the "master gland," it regulates various hormones and coordinates the endocrine system's activities.

- >> **Pineal gland:** Governs sleep patterns by secreting the hormone melatonin in response to darkness.

Each of these structures is essential for the proper functioning of the brain and contributes to the complexity of human behavior and cognitive abilities.

The control center of basic life functions

Sitting at the base of the brain is the brainstem. The brainstem is fundamental to life's bare necessities, housing the control centers for functions such as heartbeat, breathing, blood pressure, and reflexes for swallowing and vomiting. In the context of brain health, the following brainstem and related structures are particularly important:

- >> **Medulla oblongata:** Regulates vital functions, such as heart rate and respiration

- >> **Pons:** Contains nuclei that deal with sleep, respiration, swallowing, bladder control, hearing, equilibrium, taste, eye movement, facial expressions, and posture

- >> **Midbrain (Mesencephalon):** Plays a role with numerous inputs and outputs carrying information about vision, hearing, eye movement, and body movement

- >> **Reticular formation:** A network of neurons within the brainstem involved in regulating wakefulness and sleep-wake transitions

TIP

Although the cortical lobes, subcortical nuclei, and brainstem subdivisions are responsible for different jobs, they all work together. Just as musicians and their instruments come together in a symphony orchestra to create a harmonious performance, the various parts of the brain work in concert to orchestrate the complex symphony of human thoughts, emotions, and actions.

Getting a sense of your senses

Your senses are your window to the world, allowing you to perceive and interact with the environment. Vision, hearing, touch, taste, and smell work together to provide a complete picture of the world around you.

LOOKING AT VISION

Seeing is the dominant sense of humans, and 30 percent to 40 percent of your cerebral cortex is devoted to vision. This emphasis on sight is reflected in how you interact with the world around you — you likely rely on vision for everything from recognizing faces to driving your car to reading the words in this *For Dummies* book! The retina of your eye is actually an extension of your CNS and consists of specialized photoreceptor cells that turn light into electrical messages that the brain interprets. The messages travel as electrical signals along the optic nerve via the lateral geniculate nucleus of the thalamus to the visual cortex in the occipital lobe. This pathway enables you to perceive shapes, colors, and movements, forming the images we see.

LISTENING IN TO HEARING

The ears and the auditory system decipher sound waves from the environment (including the annoying fly buzzing in the background and the sound of your baby crying). Specialized hearing receptors in your inner ear's cochlea turn sound waves into electrical signals that the auditory nerve sends to the auditory cortex (via the thalamus) in the temporal lobe, enabling sound perception. Other sensory receptors inside your semicircular canals — three interconnected tubes adjacent to your cochlear — detect and transmit information about balance and spatial orientation.

GETTING A FEEL FOR TOUCH, SMELL, AND TASTE

Smell and taste are closely linked, with olfactory receptors in your nose detecting airborne chemicals, and taste buds on your tongue responding to dissolved substances, contributing to flavor, and warning you about environmental hazards (or the smell of roses!). Your somatosensory system mediates touch — a division of the PNS — where receptors in the skin respond to various stimuli such as pressure, vibration, temperature, and pain. These receptors convert physical stimuli into electrical signals transmitted via the PNS to the somatosensory cortex in the parietal lobes.

Similar receptors for pressure, vibration, temperature, and pain also transmit signals from your internal organs signaling to your brain that you're hungry, have a full bladder, or your heart is beating fast. The sense of "feelings" inside your body is known as *interception*.

Exploring the peripheral nervous system (PNS)

The peripheral nervous system (PNS) is an extensive network that connects the CNS to the rest of the body. It acts as a messenger service, relaying sensory information from the body back to the brain for processing, and delivering motor control commands from the brain to various body parts. This system ensures that the body responds appropriately to internal and external environmental changes.

Sensory and motor control

Within the PNS, motor control is managed by motor neurons, which send signals from the brain to muscles, instructing them to contract or relax to move. Sensory input is handled by sensory neurons, which carry data from sensory receptors that detect stimuli, such as touch, temperature, pain, and body position, to the brain. Sensory receptors are found throughout your body, skin, internal organs, joints, and muscles.

Counting the cranial nerves

The cranial nerves are a set of twelve nerves that originate directly from the brain and provide motor and sensory innervation mainly to the structures within the head and neck. Even though the cranial nerves originate in CNS, their main function is to connect the brain to various parts of the body, including the head, neck, and visceral organs, which qualifies them as PNS components. Each cranial nerve is numbered and named for its main function, ranging from transmitting visual information from the eyes (optic nerve) to controlling facial muscles (facial nerve) and regulating internal organs (the very famous) vagus nerve.

Deciphering the autonomic nervous system (ANS)

The ANS is the division of the PNS that regulates those body functions you don't need to think about, including your heart rate, breathing, digestion, hormone release, blood vessel constriction, and so on. The ANS consists of two main divisions: the sympathetic and parasympathetic nervous systems, which work in partnership dialing up and down to maintain your body's homeostasis (see Figure 2-5).

>> **The sympathetic nervous system (SNS),** known for its "fight or flight" response, is not exclusively triggered by imminent danger. Instead, it prepares the body for action. Actions range from ordinary tasks to thrilling events such as anticipating a Taylor Swift concert, preparing for a gold medal Olympic race,

or just raising your blood pressure so you don't faint when you stand up! By increasing your heart rate, releasing stores of energy, and directing blood to the muscles, your sympathetic nervous system prepares you for a wide range of challenges and opportunities, not just threats. This division also has a strong link to the endocrine system, notably via inputs to the adrenal glands, which secrete adrenaline, noradrenaline, and cortisol when needed.

>> **The parasympathetic nervous system (PSNS)** is called the "rest and digest" system. It conserves energy as it slows the heart rate, increases intestinal and gland activity, and relaxes sphincter muscles in the gastrointestinal tract. This division helps to promote a state of calmness, facilitating digestion and recovery.

The relationship between the SNS and PSNS is often likened to a seesaw, where an increase in activity by one system is balanced by a decrease from the other.

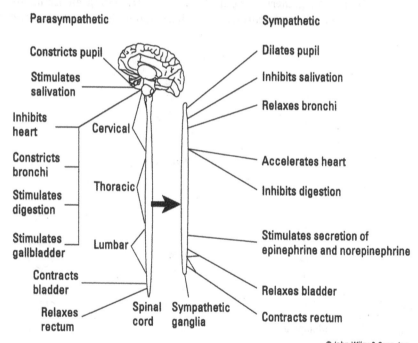

FIGURE 2-5: Divisions of the autonomic nervous system.

© John Wiley & Sons, Inc.

TIP

Adrenaline and noradrenaline are known in the United States as epinephrine and norepinephrine, respectively. This difference is largely due to historical preferences and the influence of early 20th-century pharmacology.

Connecting Neurons and Synapses

I'd now like to take you on a new adventure. Beyond the visible landscape of the brain's anatomy, into the microscopic world of neurons and glial cells, the intricate building blocks of neural architecture. In this section, you read about neurons and the precise connections — synapses — between them that give rise to your brain's remarkable abilities.

Knowing about neurons

Neurons, just like other cells in your body, have a nucleus that holds their genetic blueprint and a cell body equipped with the necessary tools to synthesize proteins and molecules. (Figure 2-6 shows different types of neurons.) However, neurons are utterly distinct from other cells. They efficiently process and transmit information, gathering inputs from the surrounding environment, as well as from other cells and neurons, through a combination of electrical and chemical signals.

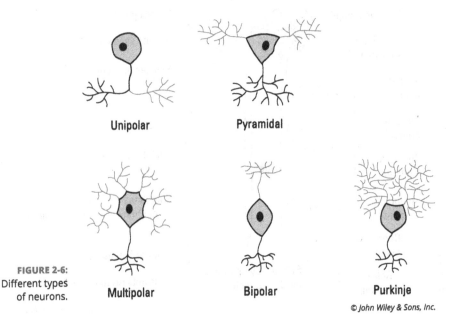

Unipolar

Pyramidal

Multipolar

Bipolar

Purkinje

FIGURE 2-6: Different types of neurons.

© John Wiley & Sons, Inc.

Here's what an individual neuron typically consists of when viewed under a microscope:

>> **Cell body:** The soma of a neuron contains the nucleus, mitochondria, and machinery for synthesizing neurotransmitters.

>> **Dendrites:** Branch-like structures that receive messages from other neurons and transmit them to the cell body.

>> **Axons:** Long, slender vine-like projections that send electrical impulses from the cell body to other neurons or muscles.

>> **Axon bulb or terminal:** The terminal or ending of an axon, where signals are sent to other neurons via the synapse.

>> **Synapse:** The small gap, known as the synaptic cleft, between two neurons where the exchange of information occurs through neurotransmitters.

Communicating with electrical impulses: The action potential

Neurons converse in two languages: electrical and chemical. The electrical language of neurons is swift and precise and is achieved by the generation of *action potentials*, often called nerve impulses or spikes. Neurons generate action potentials by integrating inputs from other neurons or sensory receptors, such as light receptors in the retina. Neurons receive both excitatory ("on") and inhibitory ("off") inputs through their dendrites, which add and subtract in a computational-like process called *synaptic integration*. The sum of "ons" and "offs" determines whether a neuron will generate action potentials and modify its own baseline firing rate.

If an action potential is triggered, it travels in one direction from the soma down the length of the axon. This process can be compared to the way electricity flows through a cable. After it reaches the axon terminal, it triggers the release of neurotransmitters into the synaptic cleft. These neurotransmitters bind to receptors on the neighboring neuron, transforming the signal into either an "on" or "off" state in the post-synaptic neuron.

Synapses: Miniature zones of communication

In their tens of billions, neurons interlink to construct your brain's intricate architecture, allowing for all the thoughts, emotions, and behaviors that define your everyday human experience. But interlinked neurons do not make direct contact with each other. Instead, there's a minuscule gap between two neurons known as a synapse, which is shown in Figure 2-7.

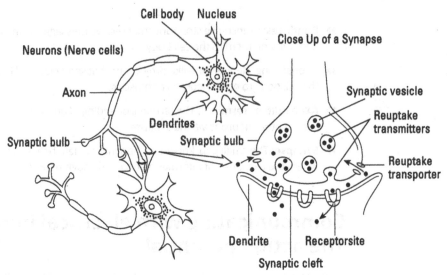

FIGURE 2-7:
Neuron
and synapse.

© John Wiley & Sons, Inc.

REMEMBER

A synapse's job is to change an electrical signal into a chemical signal. The chemical signal sends the message across the narrow synaptic split to the receiving neuron, turning it back into an electrical signal.

Here are the main components of a synapse:

>> **Presynaptic terminal or axon bulb:** The terminal end of the *pre-synaptic neuron* that releases neurotransmitters into the synapse

>> **Synaptic vesicles:** Tiny membrane bound packages within the presynaptic terminal that contain neurotransmitters

>> **Neurotransmitters:** Chemical substances that transmit signals across the synaptic cleft

>> **Synaptic cleft:** The narrow gap between the presynaptic and postsynaptic neurons

>> **Postsynaptic membrane:** The part of the neuron that receives neurotransmitters

>> **Receptors:** Protein structures on the postsynaptic membrane that bind to neurotransmitters

TECHNICAL
STUFF

Various psychoactive substances, from the caffeine in your morning coffee to therapeutic antidepressants, interact with synapses. For example, caffeine blocks receptors for a neurotransmitter that makes you feel tired, keeping you alert, while antidepressants often increase the availability of mood-regulating neurotransmitters, thereby enhancing communication between neurons.

Neurotransmitters and neuromodulators

The two major players are the neurotransmitters glutamate, which stimulates (turns "on") neural activity, and Gamma-Aminobutyric Acid (GABA), which suppresses (turns "off") neural activity. Here are some of the more well-known neurotransmitters and neuro-modulators:

>> **Glutamate** is the primary excitatory neurotransmitter found throughout the brain, involved in almost all processing from sensation to perception to cognition. Despite being integral to about 90 percent of all neural synapses, its fame hasn't quite caught up to its importance — making it perhaps the most crucial brain molecule you've never heard of!

>> **GABA** is the brain's main inhibitory ("off") neurotransmitter, helping reduce neuronal excitability. It has an important role in brain development, especially during critical periods of learning.

>> **Dopamine** is produced in several areas of the brain, including the substantia nigra and the ventral tegmental area. It plays key roles in learning, reward, motivation, and motor control. Dysregulation of dopamine levels is associated with Parkinson's disease and schizophrenia.

>> **Acetylcholine (ACh)** is found throughout the brain and body, including the nerve to muscle synapse (neuromuscular junction). Acetylcholine is involved in memory, attention, and muscle activation.

>> **Noradrenaline,** a neuromodulator mainly synthesized in the locus coeruleus of the brainstem, regulates attention and arousal. It's also made and released into the bloodstream to meet the demands of a threat or challenge.

>> **Serotonin** is produced in the raphe nuclei located along the brainstem. It is crucial for mood regulation, appetite, and sleep.

TIP

Neuromodulators are less precise and fast-acting compared to neurotransmitters. Think about them like the volume, treble, and bass knobs on a radio, fine-tuning the intensity, depth, and quality of the sound. In this analogy, neurotransmitters glutamate and GABA represent the main sound or signal being broadcast — the essential music or voice. The neuromodulators adjust how loudly or softly the brain "hears" that signal, and with what clarity and nuance, shaping the overall experience.

Receptors: Receiving the signals

Receptors in the synapse are specialized proteins embedded in the postsynaptic membrane of a synapse that bind to neurotransmitters released from the presynaptic neuron.

Think of the interaction between neurotransmitters and receptors like a key fitting into a lock. Some keys open a door. For others it's doing much more than just opening a gate — it's like initiating a sequence of operations in a sophisticated device. Likewise, when a neuromodulator binds to a metabotropic receptor, it can be compared to a key that powers up a machine, setting off a cascade of actions.

Gluing neurons together with glia

Glia comprise half the brain's cells and come in three main subtypes: astrocytes, oligodendrocytes, and microglia, which you can see in Figure 2-8. The word *glia* is Greek for "glue," because it was once assumed glia existed solely to "glue" neurons in place.

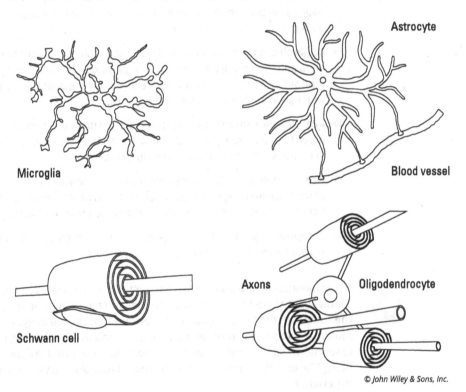

FIGURE 2-8:
Types of glia.

© John Wiley & Sons, Inc.

>> **Astrocytes,** resembling tiny stars with numerous extensions. They form the blood-brain-barrier, delivering nutrients, managing waste, and keeping neurons healthy.

>> **Microglia** are the brain's dedicated immune surveillance guards. They roam the brain tissue, searching for signs of infection or damage.

>> **Oligodendrocytes** are the brain's electricians, wrapping around axons to insulate them with a substance called myelin.

Honing in on Neuroplasticity

Neuroplasticity is the brain's remarkable ability to reorganize itself by forming new neural connections throughout life. The term encompasses a range of changes at different levels within the brain, including (but not limited to):

>> Fluctuations in action potential tempo or frequency

>> Variations in synapse efficiency, adjustments in the number or type of post-synaptic receptors, and alterations in synapse structure or shape, and the formation and removal (pruning and tuning) of synapses

>> The birth of new neurons (neurogenesis) and the programmed death of neurons (neuronal apoptosis)

>> Growth and retraction of axons and dendrites

>> Changes in the volume of grey matter (neuron cell bodies and connections) and white matter (myelinated axon tracts)

>> Reorganization of cortical maps representing sensory or motor functions

>> Changes in network strength and connectivity between brain regions

Synapse plasticity

The real magic of neuroplasticity lies in the ability of synapses to undergo modifications — *synaptic plasticity* — which is key for your brain's ability to learn and change by experience.

TIP

Imagine two neurons having a conversation. The loudness of their interaction represents synaptic efficacy — how well they communicate. This "volume" can vary; some neuronal messages are like whispers, and others are like shouts. Importantly, these communication levels are not fixed. They can change, increasing or decreasing in response to activity, which is the essence of synaptic plasticity.

Strengthening the connection over time is known as long-term potentiation (LTP), while weakening it is long-term depression (LTD). Both processes are crucial for encoding new information and adapting, making synaptic plasticity the foundation of learning and memory.

TIP

Stanford professor Carla Shatz coined the famous phrase to cleverly describe how synapses between neurons strengthen or "wire together" and prune away or "fail to link" depending on how much neural activity is present or absent. As she said, "Neurons that fire together, wire together. Neurons that are out of sync, fail to link."

Synthesizing Knowledge: How It All Works Together

Because neuroscience is so complicated, it often takes a *reductionist view*, looking closely at its smallest parts, such as neurons and synapses, because trying to understand everything at once is too hard. It's like doing a 1000-piece puzzle — you start with one piece and find where it fits before trying to combine the whole thing. Your brain's real powers come from how your neurons form networks, how robustly they connect, and how efficiently they work. When it comes to complex brain functions such as "thinking," researchers usually discuss three main brain networks:

>> **The Executive Network** is your command center for high-level thinking, decision-making, and goal-oriented tasks. It's like the CEO of the brain, directing attention, planning, and coordinating actions.

>> **The Default Mode Network (DMN)** becomes active when you daydream, reflect on the past, or imagine the future. It's involved in thinking about yourself, such as who you are, remembering your past, planning what you'll do in the future, and imagining what other people might be thinking or feeling.

>> **The Salience Network** scans for and flags important information. It decides what you should focus on and works closely with the executive network to direct your attention to the most important details in your environment.

Other networks that you may encounter as you explore brain science include:

» **The Attention Networks** two "streams" responsible for voluntary (dorsal stream) and involuntary (ventral stream) attention. They help you focus on tasks and respond to unexpected environmental stimuli.

» **The Emotional Network** processes emotions, forms memories, and helps you learn.

» **The Social Cognition Network** is engaged in understanding and navigating relationships and interactions with other people. How you understand social cues, empathize with other people's emotions, and maintain social relationships.

Modern brain imaging and analysis technologies mean researchers can watch networks in action, track how they change over development or in response to specific experiences. As you embrace the complexity of these networks, you move a small step closer to understanding the brain. From the microscale changes in synapses to the macroscale reorganization of cortical maps and network connectivity, every alteration plays a critical role in shaping your unique human experience. The trick is keeping it healthy!

IN THIS CHAPTER

» Exploring and understanding brain science research methods

» Meeting brain health professionals

» Discovering tests for assessing brain health

» Tracking your brain health

» Knowing who and when to ask for help

Chapter **3**

Measuring and Monitoring Brain Health

This chapter throws open the doors to the marvels of neuroscience and medical technology and the brilliant minds dedicated to preserving the health of your most important organ. You peek inside the laboratories where research is done to discover the powerful tools scientists use, from brain scans to artificial intelligence. And you meet the people involved in every step from the precision of genetic testing to the insights of epidemiologists.

How Scientists Study the Brain

I'm a neuroscientist who met and fell in love with the brain in the early 1990s when my Psychology 101 professor recommended we read Oliver Sacks' extraordinary book *The Man Who Mistook His Wife for a Hat*. In the book, neurologist Sacks told "inconceivably strange" tales, each one a case study of patients grappling with bewildering neurological disorders. People who navigated a world where everyday objects became unrecognizable — some even mistaking their wife for a hat (!) — while others lost parts of their memory or visual field, or possessed extraordinary talent in math or art. I was hooked. And I wasn't alone; a whole generation of students cite this book as their career inspiration.

Fields of Brain Science and Brain Health

Scientists and healthcare professionals who work in brain health draw from diverse backgrounds and specialties. You may meet a PhD student who spends their time peering at neurons in a petri dish, a neurologist working with elderly stroke patients, a psychologist who helps children with anxiety or a data scientist using machine learning to crunch information gathered from thousands of brain scans.

This list shows the wide range of disciplines and professions with a vested interest in brain science and brain health:

>> **Neuroscience** encompasses subfields such as behavioral, molecular, sensory and developmental neuroscience, which study how the brain affects behavior, the role of genes and proteins in the brain, and how the brain perceives the outside world, and develops and matures over time.

>> **Neuroimaging and neurophysiology professionals** use MRI, CT scans, and EEG to map brain structure and activity, while neurophysiologists focus on the electrical and chemical messaging within the brain.

>> **Cognitive neuroscientists and specialists** explore how mental processes such as thinking and memory are represented in the brain. They perform cognitive testing in settings such as memory clinics to diagnose and monitor conditions such as Alzheimer's disease or ADHD.

>> **Clinical neurology and psychiatry:** Neurologists diagnose and treat neurological disorders, whereas psychiatrists focus on mental health disorders. Both work on the interplay between physical brain changes and mental health symptoms.

>> **Neurosurgeons** perform surgical procedures on the brain, spine, and nerves to treat a variety of conditions ranging from traumatic injuries to congenital anomalies and tumors. They are integral to managing conditions that require anatomical correction or intervention, playing a pivotal role in treating neurological disorders.

>> **Psychologists** address mental health with various specialties, including clinical psychology for therapy, and pediatric psychology for childhood conditions such as ADHD, using cognitive tests and interventions to improve mental well-being.

- >> **Public health specialists and epidemiologists** examine the incidence and distribution of brain health issues in populations to inform prevention and control strategies at a community or population level.

- >> **Neuropharmacologists** study how medications affect the nervous system and behavior, contributing to developing new treatments for neurological and psychiatric conditions.

- >> **Computational neuroscience** is a field that creates mathematical models and simulations of brain function to analyze and interpret complex brain data. This field includes AI, machine learning, and brain imaging analysis.

- >> **Neuroendocrinology and psychoneuroimmunology** These scientists study how the endocrine and immune systems interact with the brain, affecting overall health and behavior.

- >> **Rehabilitation professionals** work to restore lost brain functions and help patients recover from brain injuries or illnesses through targeted therapies.

- >> **Developmental and educational neuroscience specialists** focus on how neurodevelopmental processes affect learning and behavior in educational settings, often working with children and young adults to optimize learning strategies and support developmental challenges.

Research tools and techniques

Researchers and healthcare professionals use various methods and tools to study the brain. Some of the more common are discussed here.

Laboratory and animal research

Neuroscience and other medical and biological research often involve studying animals to gain insights into brain function and disorders, genetics, behavior, and exploratory treatments. The most studied animals include rats, mice, fruit flies, and roundworms due to their biological similarities to humans and their suitability for lab research.

WARNING

Animal research is a topic that understandably evokes strong emotions. Until there are alternatives, it remains essential to understand biological systems, including the brain, because of the structural and functional similarities between animal and human brains. Such research is critical for medical breakthroughs and is *always* conducted under strict ethical guidelines to ensure humane treatment. It is a key contributor to the betterment of human and veterinary health and medical knowledge.

Brain imaging and brain scanning

Brain imaging or brain scanning refers to the use of advanced medical technology to create images or record activity of the brain.

Various types of imaging techniques include:

>> **MRI** (Magnetic Resonance Imaging) uses powerful magnets and radio waves to produce detailed images of the brain's structures, particularly adept at revealing soft tissues.

>> **fMRI** (Functional Magnetic Resonance Imaging) expands on MRI by detecting changes in blood flow to brain areas, allowing analysis of neural networks during various cognitive (thinking or sensory) tasks.

>> **CT Scans** (Computed Tomography) utilizes X-rays to quickly generate cross-sectional images of the brain, excellent for identifying bone injuries, hemorrhages, and tumors.

>> **PET** (Positron Emission Tomography) shows organ and tissue function by tracing an injectable radioactive substance. It's useful for studying metabolic processes and brain disorders.

>> **SPECT** (Single Photon Emission Computed Tomography) is similar to PET but with different agents, aiding in the assessment of brain blood flow and therefore correlates with neural activity.

>> **EEG** (Electroencephalography) measures electrical activity in the brain via electrodes on the scalp, and is used to study sleep and diagnosing conditions such as epilepsy. In contrast to MRI techniques, which tell us where something happens in the brain, EEG gives precise information about *when* something changes.

Computer-based analysis, machine learning, and AI

Researchers can decode intricate neurological patterns with unprecedented precision by applying machine learning algorithms or AI to massive datasets. Global research collectives have begun to pool data in "biobanks," accumulating vast amounts of data from thousands of people.

Biological sample analysis

This technique includes examining brain slices from laboratory animals or observing neurons in culture dishes, or the analysis of blood, urine, or other samples.

Clinical and neuropsychological assessment

Involves evaluating patients with cognitive tests and behavioral assessments to diagnose and understand neurological disorders. The various types of testing is covered later in this chapter.

Population-based studies and epidemiology

These studies delve into the patterns and causes of health or disease across different groups of people. This research helps to identify risk factors and to develop strategies for disease prevention and control, ultimately guiding public health policies and interventions.

Study Design and Levels of Evidence

Imagine you're trying to design a robust study to test whether apples help improve memory in older men. You must track their memory over time while accounting for other variables like diet, exercise, and health. The challenge lies in eliminating biases and isolating the effect of apples, requiring careful and systematic planning.

Here's an overview of the standard types of study design with some fictitious examples of what they may be testing.

>> **Case report:** A detailed presentation of a single patient's situation, covering their symptoms, diagnosis, treatment, and follow-up. For example, a case report may describe the progression of a rare form of dementia in a woman under 55, offering insights into potential genetic risk factors for early-onset dementia.

>> **Case series:** Similar to case reports, a group of patients with similar conditions are observed here. A neurologist may compile a case series to document the effects of a new migraine medication for teenagers.

>> **Observational studies:** These are purely about observing outcomes without any intervention. For instance, studying the natural progression of walking speed in a group of elderly men newly diagnosed with Parkinson's disease.

>> **Experimental studies:** In contrast to observational studies, these involve active intervention. An example may be testing a new anti-inflammatory drug in an emergency room setting to see its long-term effects on people presenting with a traumatic brain injury.

>> **Case-control studies:** These retrospective studies look back in time to compare two groups: those with a condition (such as stroke) and those without, to see if there was different exposure to risk factors (such as the oral contraceptive pill), measured by a statistical calculation called an *odds ratio*.

>> **Retrospective cohort:** Analyzes past data to see if exposure to a risk factor, such as head injuries by playing professional rugby, correlates with an outcome, such as the development of chronic traumatic encephalopathy (CTE) after retirement from professional sport.

>> **Prospective cohort:** Recruits people (sometimes hundreds from birth) before any outcome has occurred and follows them over time (sometimes their entire lives), assessing various factors such as childhood trauma, diet, or years of schooling and their impact on brain health as they age.

>> **Clinical trials:** These involve a sequence of phases testing new treatments or interventions in humans, often starting with small-scale safety trials and moving to large-scale efficacy and safety studies.

>> **Randomized controlled trials (RCTs):** Considered the gold standard, RCTs randomly assign participants to receive either the new intervention or a control, such as a placebo, to objectively measure treatment efficacy. An example is comparing the effects of a new cognitive-behavioral therapy regimen to standard care in patients with post-stroke depression.

In the world of brain health research (and health and medicine in general), not all evidence is created equal. What is known as *evidence-based medicine* prioritizes the highest-quality data, with RCTs leading the pack. However, RCTs aren't always possible. That's why there are meta-analyses and systematic reviews, which combine many similar studies into one data analysis that can often show patterns and answers that separate studies can't.

Navigating the Maze of Brain Health Assessments

Understanding the health of your brain is much like putting together an intricate puzzle. Each piece represents a different test or assessment, and when combined, they form a comprehensive picture of your brain's well-being. In this section, you read about some assessments or tests used to gauge brain health. Knowing more can help you make informed decisions about your own health or that of your loved ones.

Where to begin

In many countries, the pathway to address brain health concerns starts with a visit to your primary care physician, also known as a family doctor or general practitioner (GP). Your doctor (hopefully!) asks questions, listens carefully to your answers, and if necessary, orders tests or refers you to the appropriate specialist. In some parts of the world, you can head directly to a specialist or clinic without a referral.

TIP

Finding a family doctor is a proactive step toward maintaining your overall health. This step is especially important for men, who are sometimes more hesitant to seek medical care, or unlike many women, don't have a regular healthcare provider. If you don't have a regular doctor, you should ask family or friends living in your area who they see. You can also get a list of doctors in your area from your local health department or insurance company.

The types of tests to assess brain health

Evaluating brain health encompasses a broad range of assessments designed to diagnose and understand various cognitive, developmental, and psychological conditions across all age groups. The type of testing depends on the concerns you or your loved one may have.

Examples of brain health assessments include,

>> **Patient history** is taking a comprehensive patient history, which is a fundamental part of assessing brain health, involving a detailed discussion of symptoms, medical history, and family history of diseases. A neurologist, for example, may uncover a pattern of headaches in a patient's history that leads to a diagnosis of migraines.

>> **Physical and neurological examinations** are when a doctor checks for balance, coordination, and reflexes. A pediatrician may check a child's reflexes, such as the patella reflect or "knee-jerk" reflex, to ensure proper neurological development.

>> **Brain imaging and recording** is useful for diagnosing and monitoring neurological conditions, a real-world example is the use of a fmri to map brain activity by detecting changes associated with blood flow, and especially useful in pre-surgical planning for epilepsy patients.

>> **Cognitive and neuropsychological assessments** help identify impairments in cognitive functioning. You or a loved one may be asked to recall a list of words, a sequence of numbers, or the details of a story, both right away and after a few hours.

>> **Psychiatric and psychological evaluations** help with diagnosis and treatment plans for mental health disorders. A psychologist, for example, may use cognitive behavioral therapy (CBT) to treat a person with an anxiety disorder.

>> **Speech and language tests** can help identify areas of impairment after a stroke. For example, a speech-language pathologist may use the comprehensive aphasia test to tailor a rehabilitation program for a stroke survivor. *Aphasia* makes it hard to use and understand spoken and written words.

>> **Occupational and Activities of Daily Living (ADLs)** are crucial for creating targeted rehabilitation programs and determining levels of independence. ADLs are the basic tasks people need to do to take care of themselves, such as eating, showering, and getting dressed. For example, an occupational therapist may need to determine the level of assistance a patient with traumatic brain injury may need at home.

>> **Blood tests and genetic testing** can uncover underlying causes of neurological disorders. For instance, a patient with unexplained tingling in their hands may have a blood test revealing high levels of vitamin b12 deficiency, pointing to a possible neuropathy.

>> **Mental health screening** can be the first step in recognizing the need for further psychological assistance. The Edinburgh Postnatal Depression Scale (EPDS), for example, is a list of ten questions that help doctors figure out which new moms are at risk of postpartum depression.

>> **Sleep studies** help diagnose sleep disorders that can affect brain health. A person complaining of daytime fatigue and loud snoring may undergo a sleep study, resulting in a diagnosis of obstructive sleep apnea.

>> **Clinical trials** test new treatments in a controlled environment. A recent example is the clinical trials for the drug aducanumab, which included patients with early Alzheimer's disease to determine if the drug can reduce cognitive decline.

COGNITIVE TEST BATTERY

A cognitive test battery is a group of tests designed to assess brain function. When several tests are combined, they form a "battery" and give a broad picture of a person's cognitive performance. Some common tests and tasks involved include:

- **Mental speed and accuracy:** Decode a message where symbols replace letters or numbers.

- **Verbal (word) recall:** Memorize and recall a grocery list.

- **Mathematical working memory:** Solve a simple mathematical equation but simultaneously remember the solution of the previous equation.

- **Emotion recognition:** Name emotions from photos of faces, for example, sadness, happiness, fear, anger, disgust, or surprise.

- **Spatial visualization:** Rotate a complex 3D object in your mind's eye.

Keeping track of your own health

Thanks to technological progress and a better understanding of neurobiology, taking proactive care of your brain health is becoming a more realistic goal for those who are keen. With the right tools and information, you can make informed decisions about your health and wellbeing.

You already made a good start by picking up this book!

Technology and wearables

Wearables such as smartwatches and fitness trackers that can monitor your physical activity, sleep patterns, heart rate, and even stress levels. These devices use sensors to track your daily routines and can provide insights into your overall well-being, which can indirectly relate to your brain health.

Listening to friends and family

Sometimes, those closest to you may notice changes in your personality, behavior or cognitive functions before you do. Similarly, you may notice a close family showing subtle signs that worry you before they notice themselves.

Know thyself

Finally, self-awareness is a crucial aspect of tracking your brain health. Here are some questions to ask yourself that may help you consider your current brain health status:

>> Can you recall instances from the past week where your memory has notably aided or hindered you in your daily activities?

>> Are there any noticeable changes in your attention span or concentration when performing daily tasks compared to previous months or years?

>> Reflect on a recent problem you solved; how did you approach it, and were you satisfied with the process and outcome?

>> How would you rate your current stress levels, and what are the primary sources contributing to your stress?

>> On a scale of one to ten, how emotionally balanced have you felt over the past month, and what events or circumstances have influenced this?

>> Review your journal or diary entries from the past month; what patterns can you observe in your mental states and activities, and how do they align with your perception of your brain health and well-being?

IN THIS CHAPTER

» **Exploring neurodevelopmental disorders**

» **Looking at mood disorders**

» **Addressing brain injuries**

» **Understanding neurodegenerative diseases**

» **Recognizing non-diagnostic brain issues**

Chapter **4**

Examining Brain Health Disorders and Diseases

I n this chapter, you explore brain disorders, diseases, diversity, their symptoms, treatments, and a little about their underlying neurobiology. While this *For Dummies* book offers guidance to enhance your overall brain health and well-being, I want to acknowledge that such measures may not influence the risk of certain conditions developing or improving. Many disorders and diseases are shaped by genetics, chance, or terribly bad luck. That said, for other conditions, you have actionable steps that you can take to reduce your risk or improve your symptoms. Remember, health is not just about avoiding illness; it's also about maximizing each person's brain health regardless of diagnosis.

REMEMBER

Discriminatory or demeaning descriptions of people with disabilities are becoming less common. But words such as "victim" or "sufferer" still perpetuate harmful stereotypes. So, when talking to people about disorders, consider using first-persona phrases such as, "person with autism' instead of "autistic person," or "child with dyslexia" instead of "dyslexic child." And if you don't know, then ask!

Receiving a Diagnosis

When it comes to neurodevelopmental conditions, mood disorders, neurological problems and degenerative disease, diagnosis is often the first step towards support.

The Diagnostic and Statistical Manual of Mental Disorders (DSM) is the standard mental disorder classification worldwide. The current fifth edition (DSM-5) categorizes brain health symptoms, disorders, and diseases by number. Diagnoses are typically carefully made by specialists who use a combination of observations and assessments to identify these conditions.

REMEMBER

The language you might hear used to discuss these neurodevelopmental disorders has shifted in the past few decades. They are no longer solely defined as disabilities or diseases. Instead, there's a growing acknowledgment of *neurodivergence* — a term that appreciates these conditions as variations in how brains work.

Understanding Neurodevelopmental Disorders

Neurodevelopmental disorders are conditions where the typical wiring of the brain and nervous system is altered during brain development, either while growing in the womb, or during the first two years of life. They affect how the brain develops in childhood and adulthood.

Attention Deficit Hyperactivity Disorder (ADHD)

ADHD is a common neurodevelopmental condition often identified in childhood and frequently carries into adulthood. In Australia, around 6 to 10 percent of children have ADHD. Boys are three times more likely than girls to be told they have ADHD. This doesn't mean girls are less prone to the illness. Instead, one possibility is that ADHD symptoms in girls differ.

Symptoms and diagnosis

According to the online resource and support ADDitude, ADHD presents a range of symptoms that can be categorized into two distinct types, each with its own set of challenges for children and adults:

>> **Inattentive ADHD symptoms** include difficulty completing tasks, procrastination, distractibility, disorganization, and forgetfulness.

>> **Hyperactive ADHD** traits include excessive fidgeting or wriggling, persistent talking, impulsivity, constant need for stimulation, and preference for immediate rewards.

For example, a child with ADHD may find it hard to focus on their homework for long periods or may frequently jump from task to task. Whereas an adult with ADHD may struggle being on time and this may have negative consequences for their career.

Neurobiology of ADHD

Attention is a complex cognitive process that allows us to tune into specific information from our environment while tuning out of other stimuli. At the core of attentional processes is the prefrontal cortex (PFC), which acts as the conductor, directing your focus. Also involved are the neurotransmitters such as dopamine and noradrenaline that signal to the PFC to dial up or dial down its neural activity. The right balance of "loud" versus "quiet" neural activity enables you to organize your thoughts, prioritize tasks, and keep track of time.

In ADHD, this attention system operates differently. The PFC is less efficient due to variations in neurotransmitter activity. It's like having a less responsive conductor or instruments in an orchestra that ignore the conductor altogether and continue playing too loudly.

Treatment options for ADHD

Managing ADHD often requires a multifaceted approach.

>> **Educational programs** can help children develop organization and study skills.

>> **Behavioral therapy** works to reinforce positive behaviors.

>> **Medication** that acts on neurotransmitters that help regulate attention and impulsivity.

>> **Supportive measures,** such as a structured routine and clear expectations, can also be beneficial. Imagine a classroom where a teacher provides a clear, color-coded schedule — this can be a great help for a child with ADHD.

Autism Spectrum Disorder

Autism Spectrum Disorder (ASD) is a developmental condition that affects com-munication, behavior, and social interaction. Globally rates vary, which most likely reflect differences in diagnoses and reporting, but it's estimated that one in 100 people are on the autism spectrum. About three to four times as many males than females have a diagnosis. This ratio is a result of both biological differences and gender-based diagnostic criteria that may overlook autism in girls.

Symptoms and diagnosis

According to the CDC, signs and symptoms of ASD include:

>> Problems with social communication, such as not being able to read body language or hold a two-way talk

>> Repeated actions and sticking to habits; feeling upset when small things change

>> Focusing very hard on certain hobbies and interests, often knowing a lot about them

>> Sensory sensitivities, such as not liking certain sounds, smells, or lights

Neurobiology of ASD

The neurobiology of ASD involves complex interactions between genes, brain structure, and function. But there is no way to scan someone's brain and diagnose them with autism based on obvious differences. Instead, ASD is characterized by subtle differences in network connectivity and processing, especially in regions that process information about social cues.

Both environmental factors and dozens of different genes contribute to ASD risk. Some research suggests alterations in neurotransmitters and synaptic pathways emerge very early in brain development, when the baby is still in utero. Early neurogenesis (neuron cell birth) and neuron migration can have major effects on a wide range of symptoms.

Treatment options for ASD

REMEMBER

Living with ASD comes with a distinct set of challenges, but many children and adults have unique strengths and perspectives. Some people with ASD have exceptional memory, attention to detail, and expertise in their areas of interest. With understanding and tailored support, people on the autism spectrum can lead fulfilling and successful lives.

Dyslexia

Dyslexia is a specific learning disorder with a neurological basis. It is best characterized as a persistent difficulty with reading and spelling. Whereas one in five children struggle with literacy at school, about one in ten people meet the criteria of dyslexia. In a school setting, it seems to be more visible in boys, which results in earlier and more frequent identification. Dyslexia can be a problem for a person their whole life, even if they master language and literacy skills and get good, evidence-based teaching in school.

Symptoms and diagnosis

According to the Australian Dyslexia Association, common signs of dyslexia include:

» Problems learning the letter sounds for reading (decoding) and spelling (encoding)

» Difficulty in reading single words, such as on flash cards and in lists (decoding)

» Lack of accuracy and fluency when attempting to read (and decode)

» Poor spelling

» Poor visual gestalt/coding (orthographic coding)

Dyscalculia is a learning difficulty associated with math, characterized by trouble understanding numbers and mathematical concepts, while dysgraphia is a learning disability that affects writing abilities, including handwriting, spelling, and organizing ideas. Both dyscalculia and dysgraphia can also occur alongside dyslexia, indicating a broader spectrum of learning challenges.

Neurobiology of dyslexia

Brain imaging studies have identified what's known as the "reading network" in the human brain. Three major brain circuits are involved that include the left-hemisphere language centers. In fMRI brain scans of children and adults with dyslexia, a commonly observed difference is the reduced activity or "under activation" of the reading network.

Treatment options for dyslexia

Because dyslexia runs in families, it has a strong genetic basis. But like any neurodevelopmental disorder, that does not mean children can never learn to read. Early intervention is key with approaches to managing dyslexia based in the classroom and tailored to each child's needs such as:

>> Explicit instruction in phonemic awareness and phonics

>> Multisensory teaching methods to reinforce learning

>> Access to technology, such as text-to-speech and spell-checkers

>> Adjustments in teaching methods and materials

Tourette Syndrome

Tourette Syndrome (TS) is a neurological disorder characterized by tics — sudden twitches, movements, or sounds that people do repeatedly. Estimates are that TS affects about one percent of school-aged children, and boys are three to four times more likely to be diagnosed than girls. People with TS say that having a tic is like having an itch or having to sneeze. Even if you try to hold back, you'll probably scratch or sneeze at some point. This action makes you feel a little better until the urge comes back again.

Symptoms and diagnosis

Tic disorders usually start in childhood, and for lots of young people their tics decrease during adolescence and early adulthood, and sometimes disappear entirely. However, many people with TS experience tics into adulthood and, in some cases worsen. Tics sometimes increase when the person is anxious or excited or appear for no reason whatsoever.

WARNING

The media portrays people with TS as involuntarily shouting swear words (*coprolalia*) or repeating others' words (*echolalia*), yet these symptoms are infrequent and not necessary for TS diagnosis.

A person is diagnosed with TS based on their history of these tics. The hallmark symptoms of Tourette Syndrome include:

>> Multiple motor tics, such as blinking, shrugging, or jerking movements.

>> One or more vocal tics, which can include sounds like throat clearing, grunting, or more complex vocalizations.

Neurobiology of Tourette Syndrome

Deep under the surface of the cortex is a group of nuclei called the basal ganglia. This group of structures are involved in controlling and storing movements and learned automated motor skills (such as riding a bike). TS involves dysregulation within basal ganglia circuits and their connections to other brain areas. Some evidence suggests that changes in the brain's dopamine system may lead to the hyperexcitability of neurons in the basal ganglia. The over-active neurons trigger the involuntary tic movements and vocalizations. The exact causes of the dysregulation are uncertain. But data shows some children are more likely to develop tics following streptococcal throat or skin infections.

Treatment options for Tourette Syndrome

Specific treatment for tics is often unnecessary, especially if they don't disrupt day-to-day life. However, when tics are intrusive, therapies or medications may be advised. Some pediatricians suggest a watchful-waiting approach for tics that are benign, encouraging parents to disregard them rather than respond, as they're usually more awkward than harmful.

TS is often individualized and may include:

» Watchful waiting

» Behavioral therapy to manage tics

» Medication to help control severe tics when they interfere with school, for example

» Education and supportive therapies to assist with co-occurring conditions such as ADHD and OCD, which are common in individuals with TS

Living with TS can present challenges, especially in some social situations. However, there is a strong tendency for children with TS to show enhanced emotional empathy and creativity. Most people with TS lead productive and happy lives.

Managing Mood and Mental Health Disorders

Mood and mental health disorders encompass a range of conditions that profoundly affect how you feel (*emotions*), your thinking (*cognition*), and behavior. In this section you read about anxiety, depression, bipolar disorder, schizophrenia, PTSD, and OCD. These are grouped together because they all involve significant alterations in mood, thought patterns, and behavior. They're also thought to emerge from a mix of genetic, environmental, and psychological factors. Often, the treatments for them overlap.

Anxiety

Anxiety is a common mental health condition, which is characterized by excessive and prolonged worry and fear. Everyone worries from time to time, but worrying is a quick, easily resolved thought, while anxiety is accompanied by a physical response and interferes with someone's daily life. According to the World Health Organization (WHO) anxiety disorders are widespread. About four percent of the world's population experience anxiety disorders but only a quarter of those receive treatment.

Symptoms and diagnosis

Anxiety can be subdivided into: generalized anxiety disorder, social phobias, specific phobias, and panic disorders. Often anxiety disorders go hand-in-hand with other mental health issues such as clinical depression, and they may exacerbate risk factors such as social isolation.

Signs and symptoms of anxiety can include:

>> Feeling very worried or anxious most of the time

>> Finding it difficult to calm down or unable to control your anxious thoughts or worries

>> Feeling tired easily and sleep disturbances

>> Difficulty concentrating or mind going blank

>> Muscle tension

If you're not sure if you are experiencing anxiety, you can find useful online screening tools, which can help you determine if your worries will go away on their own or if you need more help.

TIP

The Black Dog Institute for mental health research in Australia states, "Feeling anxious is one way our bodies keep us safe from danger. But sometimes we can become overly worried and if it affects daily life, it may be an anxiety disorder."

Neurobiology of anxiety

Anxiety involves brain networks that process threats and regulate emotions, triggering a "fight or flight" response. Normally, the prefrontal cortex (PFC) helps modulate fear, but anxiety often arises when there's a miscommunication between the PFC and the amygdala, the brain's fear center. One idea is the excessive exposure to stress hormones make the fear brain networks "over-responsive," and it becomes hard to differentiate between innocuous challenges and dangerous threats. In a sense, everything becomes a threat.

Treatment options for anxiety

Certain drugs and cognitive-behavioral therapies try to regulate brain circuits and neurotransmitter levels to relieve anxiety symptoms. Neuroscience research and brain imaging studies are providing new insights into these complicated systems and enabling the development of tailored anxiety disorder treatments.

Three broad categories of treatment for anxiety include:

>> Psychological treatments or talking therapies.

>> Medication may be prescribed after a comprehensive health assessment and under a doctor's supervision.

>> Self-help and lifestyle treatments include exercise, nutritional adjustments, meditation, yoga, and relaxation techniques.

Depression

Depression is a commonly experienced mental health condition characterized by persistent sadness and a lack of interest in daily activities. It differs from temporary feelings of sadness, which are short-lived and often have a clear cause. The WHO reports depression affects 3.8 percent of the population, including five percent of adults (four percent males, six percent women) and 5.7 percent of those over 60. However, less than half of those affected receive treatments, partly due to diagnosis challenges and social stigma.

TIP

Australia's Black Dog Institute says, "Knowing about the causes and risk factors for depression can help you understand why depression occurs and how to deal with it. It's important to emphasize that depression is not a sign of personal weakness, failure, or 'all in the mind'."

Symptoms and diagnosis

Depression comes in many forms (or, as I like to say, in many shades of blue), including major depressive disorder, perinatal depression (occurring during pregnancy and the postnatal period), or it can co-occur with anxiety disorders and other mental health conditions.

Symptoms of depression often include:

» Persistent sadness or low mood almost every day

» Loss of interest in activities once enjoyed

» Fatigue or low energy and sleep disturbances

» Changes in appetite or weight

» Feelings of worthlessness or excessive guilt, difficulty thinking, concentrating, and making decisions

» Thoughts of death or suicide

Neurobiology of depression

Risk factors for depression span biological, psychological, and social domains, highlighting the biopsychosocial model of mental health. Genetic predispositions, neurochemical imbalances, and personality factors such as neuroticism may interact with life experiences such as bereavement, prolonged stress, or abuse, as well as cognitive patterns such as rumination, to influence an individual's vulnerability to depression.

Prolonged stress is thought to be a major factor. It is sometimes said that nature (in the form of genes, hormones, inflammation, personality, social support, or biological sex) loads the bullet and stress fires the gun.

Treatment options for depression

Treatment for depression typically falls into three main categories:

» **Psychological treatments:** CBT and other talking therapies work to change negative thought patterns and improve coping mechanisms.

» **Medication:** Antidepressant treatment decisions are made after a thorough health assessment and should be closely monitored by healthcare professionals. In many countries, medication is *not* the first-line treatment for mild to moderate depression.

» **Lifestyle changes:** Regular exercise, a healthy balanced diet, plenty of sleep, and stress reduction strategies can support other treatment methods and contribute to overall well-being.

Bipolar disorder

Bipolar disorder is a complex psychiatric condition marked by extremes of mood, including emotional highs (mania or hypomania) and lows (depression). The WHO estimates that it affects about 45 million people worldwide or about two percent of the population. People with bipolar disorder are often untreated because they're misdiagnosed or lack access to appropriate care.

Symptoms and diagnosis

Bipolar disorder manifests in several forms, including Bipolar I, Bipolar II, and Cyclothymic Disorder, each with distinct patterns of mood swings. People with Bipolar I disorder may not suffer depressed episodes and instead experience more intense manias. Whereas people with Bipolar II also have sad episodes in addition to a milder high (hypomania). Cyclothymic disorder is a milder form of bipolar disorder, involving frequent mood swings between mild highs (hypomania) and mild lows (depression).

Symptoms include:

>> Periods of excessively elevated mood, energy, and frenetic activity (mania)

>> Episodes of feeling sad, hopeless, or losing interest in most activities (depressive episode)

>> Changes in sleep patterns, activity levels, and behavior

Early diagnosis can be challenging but is essential for managing the condition. A comprehensive assessment by a mental health professional such as a psychiatrist is critical to help people get treatment.

Neurobiology of bipolar disorder

The causes of bipolar disorder involve a mix of genetics, neurotransmitter imbalances, and environmental stressors, fitting within the biopsychosocial framework. Bipolar disorder is frequently inherited, with genetic factors accounting for approximately 80 percent of the cause of the condition. One way to think about risk is that genes predispose some people to bipolar disorder, which triggered by factors such as extreme stress or life events. Brain imaging studies have shown structural and functional changes in areas related to emotion regulation and impulse control, such as the prefrontal cortex and the amygdala.

Treatment options for bipolar disorder

Customized treatment regimens include medicine, psychotherapy, and lifestyle modifications to provide the best possible results. Effective management of bipolar disorder typically includes:

>> Medication such as antipsychotics, antidepressants, and mood stabilizers are frequently used to manage mood swings.

>> Psychotherapy or talking therapies including CBT, family-focused therapy, and psychoeducation.

>> Lifestyle changes to preserve emotional stability, regular exercise, good sleep hygiene, and routines and schedules are also prescribed.

Schizophrenia

Schizophrenia is a severe psychiatric disorder that affects how a person thinks, feels, and behaves. Common experiences include hallucinations, delusions, and disorganized thinking. According to WHO, its estimated to affect 20 million people worldwide. In Australia, schizophrenia affects around 2.4 per 1000 people. Symptoms of schizophrenia usually develop in the late teens or early 20s — though they can appear later in life, especially in women.

Symptoms and diagnosis

One of the main symptoms of schizophrenia is psychosis. A person experiencing psychosis finds it hard to tell what is real from what isn't. Psychosis is usually experienced in episodes — short periods of intense symptoms. Each person can experience different kinds of symptoms, and the symptoms can change from one attack to the next.

Two or more of the following must happen to a person for at least a few months in order to be diagnosed with schizophrenia:

>> Delusions are false ideas that can't be changed, even if proof is shown.

>> People who hallucinate may hear, see, or feel things that aren't there.

>> Disorganized thinking including speech and thoughts that aren't normal or are jumbled.

>> Disorganized behaviors include actions that are out of the ordinary, wrong, or extreme.

Neurobiology of schizophrenia

Schizophrenia has more than one cause. Because genes play a big role in the chance of getting schizophrenia, people who have a family history of it are more likely to get it themselves. Some factors make the chances of getting schizophrenia higher. For example, differences in a person's brain chemistry, stressful social situations, and trauma (especially as a child). There's also a link between substance use and schizophrenia, but this relationship is complex. Some unexpected factors influence the development of the condition including, being born in the winter or living in an urban versus countryside setting.

Treatment options for schizophrenia

Treatment for schizophrenia is lifelong and often involves a combination of antipsychotic medications, which are the cornerstone of managing symptoms, and psychosocial therapies. Some drugs work better in some people than others, and the reasons remain unclear.

Psychosocial interventions, including psychotherapy, social skills training, and vocational rehabilitation, are essential for improving functioning and quality of life. Managing lifestyle factors, such as stress levels, diet, and exercise, also plays a role in treatment plans. Integrated care that includes medication, therapy, and social support offers the best prognosis for those living with schizophrenia.

Post-Traumatic Stress Disorder (PTSD)

PTSD is a severe mental health condition triggered by experiencing or witnessing a traumatic event. Many different harmful or life-threatening events may cause PTSD. For example, being in in a car crash, being raped, being in a natural disaster, experiencing violence, or seeing other people hurt or killed, or any event in which you fear for your life.

The WHO indicates PTSD affects approximately 3.6 percent of the global population in any given year, with higher rates in groups of people exposed to severe conflict or war. In countries such as Australia, up to 12 percent of people will experience PTSD in their lifetime, with most among first responders (for example, police or paramedics) and military personnel.

REMEMBER

Acknowledge that PTSD is a response to trauma or an event beyond your control. PTSD is not a sign of personal weakness.

Symptoms and diagnosis

Common experiences of PTSD include reliving the traumatic event through flash-backs, nightmares, and distress at reminders of the incident, often accompanied by physical reactions such as pain or shaking.

Flashbacks are vivid memories of traumatic events that feel like they're happening right now. Flashbacks can be like viewing a video, although they don't always entail images or remembering experiences. Some people experience:

>> Visions, sounds, scents, and tastes related to the trauma, physical sensations such as pain or pressure, and emotions experienced during the trauma.

>> Heightened alertness or hypervigilance, resulting in panic, irritability, trouble sleeping, difficulty concentrating, and a heightened startle response.

>> Individuals may experience intense distress at real or symbolic reminders of the trauma, persistent fear, and a feeling of detachment from others.

Neurobiology of PTSD

PTSD arises from a complex interplay between the brain's fear response networks, personal history, and the severity of the traumatic exposure. Brain imaging studies have shown alterations in the amygdala, hippocampus, and prefrontal cortex, which are associated with a heightened fear response and memory processing. The condition is linked with prolonged exposure to stress hormones such as cortisol, which can lead to changes in brain function and structure.

Treatment options for PTSD

Effective treatments for PTSD may include:

>> **Psychological therapies:** Trauma-focused CBT, Eye Movement Desensitization and Reprocessing (EMDR), and Exposure Therapy are common methods. These therapies help process the trauma, reduce symptoms, and teach coping strategies.

>> **Medication:** While not always the first line of treatment, SSRIs and SNRIs may be prescribed to manage symptoms, particularly when accompanied by careful medical supervision.

>> **Lifestyle modifications:** Strategies such as regular physical activity, sufficient sleep, and mindfulness practices can bolster resilience and support recovery alongside clinical treatments.

Studies of traumatic events show people are resilient. While up to two out of three people will suffer at least one traumatic event in their lifetime, most (70 percent) showing resilience, some people take time to recover, and even fewer develop PTSD.

Navigating Neurological Problems

Neurological problems, such as migraines and epilepsy, are conditions that directly impact the brain. For example, migraines manifest as severe headaches alongside symptoms such as sensitivity to light, while epilepsy is characterized by recurrent, unprovoked seizures.

Migraine

Migraine is a neurological condition often characterized by intense, debilitating headaches. Symptoms may include nausea, vomiting, difficulty speaking, numbness or tingling, and sensitivity to light and sound. Migraine is listed as the sixth most disabling disorder globally, and the most common neurological disorder. In Australia, it is reported that migraines affect approximately 4.9 million people, or around 20 percent of the population.

Typically, migraine onset occurs during adolescence or early adulthood. They're more common in women than men, which is likely due to female sex hormones. Although they can start in childhood or adolescence, most migraine patients typically have symptoms in their 20s or 30s. They're less common after age 40, but different types of migraine afflict people at different life stages. Migraine can also run in families.

Symptoms and diagnosis

Migraine attacks can cause significant headache pain for hours to days and can be so severe that the pain is disabling. Movement typically exacerbates the pain and people also experience nausea, vomiting, and sensitivity to light, sound, and smells. After the migraine attack people report feelings ranging from exhaustion to euphoria, and often lingering fatigue and sensitivity to light and sound.

Some people experience what are known as prodromal symptoms (warning signs) up to 24 hours before the headache starts. A common warning sign for about 20 percent of people is aura. *Aura* often affects your vision and is described as flashes of light or blind spots that move across the visual field, or like looking at a mirage or heat waves on a hot road. Other sensations include nausea, tingling on one side of the face or in an arm or leg, or difficulty speaking.

TIP

If you're uncertain about your headaches, it's always wise to chat to your doctor. Keeping a "headache diary" including symptoms, possible triggers, and their impact on work or social life can greatly assist your doctor in understanding migraine and determining the most effective treatment.

Neurobiology of migraine

Sometimes people are able to pinpoint triggers for their migraine, and in turn avoid situations that cause them. Common triggers include:

» Hormones fluctuations

» Certain foods and drinks, such as aged cheeses, red wine, processed meats, chocolate, caffeine, and artificial sweeteners

» Intense lights, sunlight, loud sounds, and strong smells

» Environmental triggers including weather shifts, altitude changes, time zone changes, and exposure to smoke or pollutants

» Stress and changing sleep patterns

Migraines begin with a spreading cortical depression — an electrical wave moving through the cortex — which manifests as aura. Another pathway involved is the trigeminal nerve system, a pain pathway in the head and face. Because aura often precedes the headache, it's thought the cortical spreading depression activates the trigeminal nerves to release pro-inflammatory substances around the brain's blood vessels and meninges. In turn, the pro-inflammatory substances induce the blood vessel dilation and inflammation that contribute to the severe pain of a migraine.

The neurotransmitter serotonin is also closely linked to migraine. Changing serotonin levels may trigger pulsating of cerebral blood vessels, adding to migraine's characteristic throbbing pain. Many migraine medications target serotonin receptors, mimicking serotonin's effects.

Treatment options for migraine

Medications are aimed at stopping symptoms and preventing future attacks. Many medications have been designed to treat migraines. Medications used to combat migraines fall into two broad categories: pain-relieving medications and preventive medications. Triptans are most commonly prescribed, and they act by binding to serotonin receptors as described previously.

Epilepsy

Epilepsy is a chronic neurological disorder marked by recurrent, unprovoked seizures due to abnormal electrical discharges in the brain. Globally, the number of people with active epilepsy (that is, continuing seizures or with the need for treatment) at a given time is between four and ten per 1000 people. People with epilepsy are at risk of accidents leading to injury or death often due to seizures that can result in falls, drowning, or burns. This risk is particularly in low- and middle-income countries when effective treatment and management of the condition are not accessible.

Symptoms and diagnosis

Seizures, the main symptom of epilepsy, can vary from person to person, from brief lapses of attention (absence seizures) to severe and prolonged convulsions. And depending who is experiencing them, they vary in their impacts on consciousness, movement, and sensation.

Epilepsy commonly shows up in childhood or adolescence, but it can occur at any age. Sometimes epilepsy runs in families, indicating a genetic component, but it also results from brain injury, stroke, or infection. That said, in about 50 percent of cases, the cause remains unknown.

Neurobiology of epilepsy

The neurobiology of epilepsy involves complex interactions within the brain's electrical system. Disruptions in this system lead to seizures. Because the causes of epilepsy are so varied, the disruptions can be caused by genetic predispositions, structural brain changes (for example, tumor), or imbalances in neurotransmitters.

Treatment of epilepsy

Treatment of epilepsy is personalized and may include medications called antiepileptic drugs, which are the mainstay in managing seizures. In some cases, surgical intervention, or dietary changes such as a ketogenic diet may be considered.

If conventional treatments fail to control seizures, some people consider medicinal cannabis. However, this option should only be considered after consulting with a specialized doctor and after exploring all other FDA-approved treatments.

Managing epilepsy effectively requires a comprehensive care approach that can minimize the frequency and severity of seizures and improve the quality of life for individuals with the condition.

Addressing Structural and Acquired Brain Disorders

In this section you read about brain health problems that involve damage or injury to the brain's structure, which in turn affect how it works, and consequently, health and behavior. Strokes are caused by disruptions of blood flow to the brain, traumatic brain injuries (TBI), and spinal cord injuries (SCI) are usually the result of a knock to the head, and brain tumors are masses of cells that grow uncontrollably. Damage to the brain or spinal cord requires a very different approach compared to other psychological or developmental brain health conditions.

Brain tumors

Brain tumors are abnormal growths of cells within the brain that can disrupt normal brain function. In Australia, the incidence of brain cancer has rates ranging between seven and nine cases per 100,000 people, although the rate is slightly higher in men than women. There are more than 40 types of brain and spinal cord tumors and they're classified based on the type of cell they start in. Gliomas are tumors that start in the glial cells of the brain and are the most common type.

Symptoms and diagnosis

Symptoms of brain tumors depend on the tumor's location and how fast its growing. Some tumors are found at a very advanced stage, others much earlier. Brain tumors may cause increased skull pressure, leading to symptoms such as morning headaches, nausea, vision changes, seizures, unconsciousness, weakness, and later, drowsiness. Brain tumor diagnosis starts with a doctor's assessment if symptoms point to a neurological issue.

Tests include:

>> Neurological checks for brain function

>> Blood tests for health and hormonal imbalances

>> MRI for detailed imaging, CT for cross-sectional views

>> Additional scans and biopsies to understand tumor growth and genetics

Tumors are graded from 1 (low-grade, slow) to 4 (high-grade, fast, likely to recur). The grading suggests how quickly the tumor may grow.

Neurobiology of brain tumors

How tumors impact the brain depends on their type, size, and location. Notably, glioblastomas, which are the most aggressive and common of malignant brain tumors, represent a significant proportion of cases and are notorious for their poor prognosis, with a five-year relative survival rate of about six percent. In contrast, another type of brain tumor, oligodendroglioma, which is characterized by specific genetic mutations has a five-year survival rate of 84 percent. The neurobiology and pathophysiology of brain tumors are complex, and such as cancer, involving a variety of genetic and molecular mechanisms that drive tumor growth and survival.

Treatment of brain tumors

Brain tumor treatment aims to remove the tumor, slow its growth, or relieve symptoms, depending on the tumor's characteristics and the patient's health. Treatment options include:

- » Surgery to remove all or part of the tumor or to relieve pressure
- » Radiation therapy to target cancer cells to reduce the tumor's size or prevent its growth
- » Chemotherapy using drugs that cross the blood-brain barrier to treat cancer cells
- » Steroids to reduce swelling in the brain
- » Palliative care to improve quality of life by managing symptoms

Given their significant impact on health (especially of children and young people), social, and economic factors, brain tumors are a focus of ongoing research and clinical trials, aiming to improve diagnosis, treatment, and survival outcomes for those affected by this challenging condition.

Traumatic brain injury (TBI)

TBI is a significant health concern globally, affecting people across all demographics, often rather unexpectedly with devastating consequences to health. Common causes of TBI include falls, motor vehicle-related collisions, domestic violence, military combat, and sports injuries. Brain injuries can range from very mild (such as concussion) to severe (such as TBI), characterized by symptoms such as headaches and dizziness, to more pronounced issues such as slurred speech and loss of consciousness.

Symptoms and diagnosis

Symptoms of TBI can vary based on severity. A mild TBI, or concussion, often results from a knock to the head or violent shaking, leading to symptoms such as headaches, confusion, dizziness, and visual disturbances. Memory loss surrounding the incident may occur.

Severe TBI may present with more alarming signs, including extended unconsciousness or amnesia. Diagnosis involves clinical evaluation, which may include neuroimaging to assess the extent of brain injury and neuropsychological tests to understand cognitive impairment.

Neurobiology of TBI, concussion, and CTE

TBI involves complex pathophysiological processes. Even a closed-head injury, for example knocking your head while wearing a cycle helmet can lead to axonal shearing, where the brain's movement inside the skull causes axons to stretch and tear. This disrupts neuron to neuron communication and can lead to cell death. Shearing of axons is a hallmark of diffuse axonal injury, which can have devastating neurological consequences.

In concussion, which is considered a mild TBI, similar mechanisms may operate on a smaller scale but can accumulate with repeated injuries, or over time, increasing the risk for conditions such as chronic traumatic encephalopathy (CTE). CTE is associated with the buildup of tau protein in the brain, which impairs neuronal function and can lead to symptoms such as memory loss, confusion, impaired judgment, and progressive dementia.

Treatment of TBI

Treatment for TBI spans emergency care to rehabilitation and long-term care planning. For milder forms such as concussion, rest and a gradual return to activities are prescribed to allow the brain to heal. Severe TBIs may require surgical intervention to alleviate pressure or repair damage. Ongoing rehabilitation, including physical, occupational, and speech therapy, supports recovery.

Stroke

Stroke is a critical health issue, striking people rather unexpectedly and with varying degrees of severity. *Stroke* occurs when the blood supply to part of the brain is interrupted or reduced, preventing brain tissue from getting oxygen and nutrients. This can lead to cell death, leaving an area called a cerebral infarct. Around the world, one in four people above the age of 25 is likely to experience a stroke at some point in their lives. Annually, more than 16 percent of strokes happen in individuals aged 15 to 49 years. For many who don't receive immediate and appropriate care, the resulting disability is devasting.

Symptoms and diagnosis

The symptoms of a stroke depend on the region of the brain affected. Quick diagnosis and treatment are critical.

People are encouraged to use the F.A.S.T test if they suspect a stroke:

>> **Face:** Check their face. Has their mouth drooped?

>> **Arms:** Can they lift both arms?

>> **Speech:** Is their speech slurred? Do they understand you?

>> **Time is critical:** If you see any of these signs call emergency services or paramedics straight away.

Facial weakness, arm weakness and difficulty with speech are the most common symptoms or signs of stroke, but they are not the only signs. People may have trouble with speech or comprehension, alongside possible dizziness and balance issues, which may lead to unexplained falls. Vision can be abruptly impaired or blurred in either one or both eyes. Severe headaches that appear suddenly or represent a change in the pattern of previous headaches can occur. There may also be trouble with swallowing.

Neurobiology of stroke

Two types of strokes are:

>> **Ischemic strokes** where blockages such as clots disrupt blood flow. This ischemia triggers a harmful cascade of cellular reactions, including excitotoxicity, where an excess of neurotransmitters causes further neuronal damage, and inflammation, which inadvertently harms healthy cells.

>> **Hemorrhagic strokes** are caused by ruptured blood vessels, leading to bleeding that directly damages brain cells and elevates intracranial pressure, impairing blood flow and potentially causing more extensive injury.

Treatment of stroke

Treatment strategies for stroke focus on restoring blood flow for ischemic stroke or controlling bleeding and reducing pressure in the brain for hemorrhagic stroke. Immediate treatment may include thrombolytic drugs to dissolve clots or surgery in certain cases. Post-stroke rehabilitation is crucial and may involve speech therapy, physiotherapy, and occupational therapy to aid recovery.

Investigating Neurodegenerative Disorders

Understanding dementia and other brain diseases of aging sheds light on the critical risk factors that influence brain health over your lifespan. By delving into the details of age-related diseases, you can understand the importance of preserving cognitive function and quality of life as we navigate the later chapters of our existence.

REMEMBER

Dementia is an umbrella term used to describe various symptoms of cognitive decline, such as forgetfulness. It is a symptom of several underlying diseases and brain disorders. Alzheimer's disease (AD) is the most common cause of dementia. Other types include vascular dementia, Lewy body dementia, and frontotemporal dementia, which is related to the shrinking of the frontal and temporal anterior lobes of the brain. Each type of dementia is classified based on its distinct pathological features, causes, and patterns of brain changes, as well as the specific symptoms it presents.

Alzheimer's disease (AD)

AD is a common neurodegenerative condition worldwide, predominantly affecting the elderly population. *AD* is characterized by progressive memory loss, cognitive decline, and personality changes.

Although it is not the cause of AD, getting older is the biggest known risk factor for the illness. Beyond the age of 65, the number of AD cases about doubles every five years. Estimates vary by country but approximately one-third of adults over 85 in the U.S. may develop AD. That said, many people do not experience dementia until they are in their 90s or older.

Women tend to be more affected by AD than men, but rates in men are catching up. Several reasons may explain this: women generally live longer, they may have different hormonal levels and genetic factors that make them more susceptible, and they're more likely to get conditions such as depression, which can increase the risk of AD.

Symptoms and diagnosis

Symptoms of dementia include:

>> A decline in memory

>> Changes in thinking skills

>> Poor judgment and reasoning skills

>> Decreased focus and attention

>> Changes in language

>> Changes in behavior

REMEMBER

Memory loss is a core symptom of dementia. Everyone forgets things sometimes, but dementia is different. It persists and advances. It may hinder work or familiar tasks. It can be hard to get home. It can lead to forgetting how to dress or bathe. Normal forgetfulness includes forgetting why you entered the kitchen or losing the car keys. However, a dementia patient may lose their car keys and forget the key's purpose.

Neurobiology of AD

AD involves the buildup of amyloid plaques and tau tangles in the brain, causing nerve cell connections to be lost and the brain tissue to shrink, particularly in areas crucial for thought and memory. This leads to changes that can be seen with the naked eye (or microscope) including brain atrophy, particularly in the cerebral cortex and hippocampus, enlargement of fluid-filled ventricles, breakdown in white matter that connects brain regions, and a decrease in brain weight.

Under a microscope, you can see:

>> Plaques from beta-amyloid protein clusters.

>> Neurofibrillary tangles of tau protein inside neurons, which interfere with neuron function and are linked to cell death.

Historically, the accumulation of beta-amyloid plaques was believed to be the primary driver of AD (they disrupted communication between neurons, triggered inflammation, leading to cell death). However, plaque load and cognitive impairment are not always linear. Some elderly individuals have a significant plaque load but show no cognitive impairment, while others may not exhibit as much plaque.

BETA-AMYLOID, TAU, AND GENETIC FACTORS IN AD

There's also debate over which comes first in the AD pathology: beta-amyloid accumulation or tau-related changes. Moreover, several high-profile clinical trials targeting beta-amyloid have failed to show significant benefits (others have shown some minor benefit), casting doubt on the centrality of plaques in AD progression.

Dementia isn't caused by a single gene, but certain genes such as Apolipoprotein E (APO-e4) on chromosome 19 can affect risk, with APO-e4 carriers possibly showing Alzheimer's symptoms earlier, although not all will develop the disease. In contrast, early onset familial Alzheimer's disease (FAD) is directly caused by mutations in specific genes (presenilin 1, presenilin 2, and the amyloid precursor protein gene) and typically manifests in middle age, with a 50 percent chance of passing it on to children.

Treatment options for AD

While there is currently no cure for AD, treatments are available to help manage symptoms. Therapeutic strategies may include medications to improve symptoms of memory decline and other cognitive abilities, as well as to manage behavioral changes. Supportive interventions focus on helping individuals and their families cope with the challenges of AD, including educational resources, support groups, and services offered by organizations such as Dementia Australia.

Parkinson's Disease (PD)

PD is a chronic and progressive movement disorder that affects approximately 10 million people worldwide. It commonly impacts individuals over the age of 60, with both incidence and prevalence rising with age. Like AD, the exact cause of PD is unknown, but a combination of genetic and environmental factors is believed to contribute.

Symptoms and Diagnosis

The primary symptoms of PD include:

>> Tremors of the hands, arms, legs, jaw, and face

>> Rigidity or stiffness of the limbs and trunk

>> Slowness of movement (bradykinesia)

>> Impaired balance and coordination, leading to difficulties in walking and a higher risk of falls

As the disease progresses, symptoms may worsen and include difficulty speaking, anxiety, depression, and cognitive impairment.

Neurobiology of PD

PD is characterized by the loss of dopamine-producing neurons in the substantia nigra, a region of the midbrain, and the presence of Lewy bodies — abnormal aggregates of protein — that develop inside nerve cells, affecting motor control and other functions.

The loss of dopaminergic neurons leads to a drop in dopamine levels, which is crucial for regulating movement and coordination. As dopamine decreases, PD symptoms begin to emerge. The presence of Lewy bodies is also associated with the symptoms of PD, although their exact role in the disease process is not fully understood. The genetic factors in PD are less well-defined than in AD, with multiple genes and environmental factors implicated.

Treatment of PD

While no cure for PD exists, treatments such as medication and surgical therapy can manage its symptoms. The most common medication is levodopa combined with carbidopa, which is converted to dopamine in the brain.

Brain stimulation treatments, such as Deep Brain Stimulation (DBS), involves surgically implanting electrodes into specific areas of the brain. The device sends electrical impulses to the brain to regulate abnormal impulses, or to affect certain cells and chemicals within the brain. For patients whose symptoms cannot be adequately managed with medication, DBS can significantly enhance quality of life.

Multiple Sclerosis (MS)

MS is a chronic inflammatory condition of the central nervous system, affecting millions worldwide. Unlike AD, MS can occur at any age, but most commonly is diagnosed in individuals between the ages of 20 and 40. It has a variety of presentations, ranging from mild to severe, and is more common in women than in men. In Australia, the prevalence of MS has also risen considerably. In 2021, 131.12 Australians per 100,000 (0.013 percent) of people lived with MS, up from 103.7 per 100,000 in 2017.

MS is characterized by the immune system abnormally attacking the protective sheath (myelin) that covers nerve fibers, causing communication problems between your brain and the rest of your body. Eventually, the disease can cause the nerves themselves to deteriorate or become permanently damaged.

Symptoms and diagnosis

Symptoms can vary widely and may include:

» Numbness, weakness, tingling or electric shocks in one or more limbs or other body parts

» Partial or complete loss of vision or double vision

» Tremor, lack of coordination, or unsteady gait

» Slurred speech, fatigue and dizziness

» Problems with bowel and bladder function

REMEMBER

MS symptoms are unpredictable and vary in intensity. While one person may experience fatigue and numbness, another may have severe vision problems and mobility impairments. Symptoms can fluctuate or steadily advance over time.

Neurobiology of MS

MS involves a process called demyelination. Myelin damage disrupts the transmission of messages within the central nervous system. This damage can lead to a range of neurological symptoms, depending on which part of the CNS is affected.

Under a microscope, you can see:

» Areas of damage (lesions) on the brain and spinal cord

» Plaques or scarring due to chronic inflammation

» Loss of myelin and, eventually, the nerves themselves

The exact cause of MS is unknown, but it's believed to be a combination of genetic susceptibility and environmental factors, such as viral infections. Vitamin D deficiency and smoking are also associated with a higher risk of developing MS.

Treatment options for MS

While there's no cure for MS, treatments can help speed recovery from attacks, modify the course of the disease and manage symptoms. These include:

>> Disease-modifying therapies (DMTs) that can reduce disease activity and progression in many people with relapsing forms of MS.

>> Corticosteroids and plasma exchange for managing relapses.

>> Physical therapy, muscle relaxants, and medications to reduce fatigue and improve mobility.

Motor Neuron Disease (MND)

Motor Neuron Disease (MND) includes a group of neurological disorders that affect motor neurons. Motor neurons innervate voluntary muscle and control activities such as speaking, walking, breathing, and swallowing. Amyotrophic Lateral Sclerosis (ALS) is the most common form of MND. MND typically manifests in adults over 40 and is slightly more prevalent in men. Globally, the incidence of MND is approximately one to two per 100,000 people annually.

MND leads to progressive weakness and wasting of muscles caused by the degeneration of motor neurons in the brain and spinal cord. The etiology of MND is not fully understood; however, it's thought to be due to a combination of genes and environmental factors.

Symptoms and diagnosis

Symptoms of MND are progressive and can include:

>> Gradual weakening of muscles, often beginning with a limb

>> Slurred speech and difficulty with swallowing

>> Muscle stiffness and cramps and progressive difficulty with movement and coordination

These symptoms vary between individuals, and some people, sadly, experience rapid progression and others having a more protracted disease course.

MND is difficult to diagnose but confirmed MND diagnosis is the first step to proper care, support, and treatment. The two main types of testing including, nerve conduction studies (NCS) examine the neurological system using nerve stimulation and muscle activity recording, while electromyography (EMG) measures muscle activity using needle electrodes.

Neurobiology of MND

MND involves loss of motor neurons. Two classes of MND can affect either: Upper motor neurons that project from the primary motor cortex down the spinal cord, and lower motor neurons that project from the spinal cord to muscles.

MND is characterized by:

» Progressive loss of motor neurons in the spinal cord and brain.

» Muscle atrophy and weakness due to lack of stimulation by affected neurons.

» Clumping of protein aggregates found inside degenerating motor neurons (most often the TDP-43 protein).

About 15 percent of cases are familial, passed down through a gene mutation, but other theories about the causes of motor neuron disease (MND) include exposure to environmental toxins and chemicals, viral infections, and immune-related damage.

Treatment of MND

There's no cure for MND, and treatment is aimed at symptom management and maintaining quality of life. Treatment strategies may include:

» Medications to slow disease progression, such as riluzole for ALS.

» Assistive technology and adaptive equipment to maintain independence.

» Multidisciplinary care teams providing physical therapy, respiratory therapy, and nutritional support.

Research into MND is advancing, with a focus on understanding the underlying pathophysiological processes and developing treatments to slow or halt the progression of the disease.

IN THIS CHAPTER

» Decoding statistics in brain health

» Weighing up risks and benefits

» Unpacking prevalence and incidence

» Assessing genetic versus lifestyle influences.

» Understanding holistic views of brain health

Chapter **5**

Calculating the Causes and Risks of Brain Health Problems

The mere mention of math may send even the bravest of you running for the hills, chased by visions of calculators, quadratic equations, and t-tests. But bear with me! Making sense of statistics and discussions of complicated concepts such as relative risk, prevalence, and percentages can be difficult when you're trying to make informed health decisions.

In this chapter, I demystify the complex world of statistical data, so you can identify your brain health risk factors with more confidence than you may have now. Beyond numbers, you look at the many pieces that interact to determine health and disease, giving you a complete picture of the forces at work behind the scenes of science.

Understanding Statistical Terms Simply

Navigating the world of health risk factors, both good and bad, can feel like a trip through a maze of hormones, lifestyle choices, and sensationalist news headlines, from flu scares to shark encounters to debating whether red meat is the best or worst thing you can eat! However, understanding the concept of *risk* is a critical step toward protecting your brain health. With the right knowledge, you can discover how to sidestep potential dangers and ease unfounded worries about implausible hazards. So, let's take a closer look at the concept of risk.

Weighing up risks and benefits

Imagine you have clinical depression and are considering switching to a new medication. Your doctor will explain the risks, such as side effects, and the benefits, like reduced depressive symptoms. To make a decision, you need to balance the severity and likelihood of side effects against the potential relief.

For example, if the drug offers significant symptom relief with minor side effects like an itchy scalp, you may find it worth trying. However, if it causes insomnia in most people and only works for a few, the risks may outweigh the benefits. Like an old-fashioned scale, risks and benefits can tip the balance toward different outcomes.

WARNING

Sometimes the decision or weight of risks is obvious. Other times it isn't. In some confusing instances, scientists and doctors haven't yet figured out if a behavior or activity is risky (that is, how heavy or light a weight is and which side of the scales to place it!). And as new data emerges from a study about a particular disease, the risk (or heaviness of a weight) often changes.

Risk is relative, so absolutely look for absolute risk!

If you happen to stumble across discussions of risk (in the newspaper, or in the pages of this book!) it is useful to know where the numbers come from and what they mean. Typically, they're calculated in the process of a meta-analysis. They're particularly useful in healthcare research to determine the effectiveness of treatments or interventions across different populations and study designs.

The statistics reported by these studies include:

>> **Relative risk** (RR) is a number showing how much the risk of something happening (such as developing a disease) in one group compares to the risk

in another group. If RR is more than 1.0, there's a higher risk in the first group compared to the second. If the RR is less than 1.0, the risk is lower. An RR of exactly 1.0 means the risks are the same in both groups. Comparing risks helps us understand the effect of a certain action or exposure.

>> **Absolute risk** is the number to *absolutely* pay attention to. It's the straightforward chance of something happening to *you*, without comparing it to anyone else. It's like saying, "Out of 100 people, X number will likely experience this." It's a direct measure of risk that applies to an individual or a specific group.

REMEMBER

Absolute risk is absolutely the most important number to focus on because it gives you a direct idea of your chances of experiencing something. For example, in this case, Mary is a 55-year-old woman in good health. According to The Framingham Heart Study, a long-term investigation aimed at uncovering factors contributing to cardiovascular disease, Mary's absolute risk of stroke over her lifetime is 21.1 percent.

Understanding the absolute risk of 21.1 percent means out of 100 women like Mary, about 21 of them would likely have a stroke over their lifetime.

Now, RR helps you compare risks between different groups. For instance, a meta-analysis published in 2009 found that women who closely follow the Mediterranean Diet had a 13 percent lower RR of stroke compared to those who didn't eat Mediterranean-style food. This factor was represented by an RR of 0.87.

Simply put, if Mary starts following the Mediterranean Diet, it could reduce her absolute risk by 13 percent of 21.1 percent. This means Mary's absolute risk of stroke could decrease from 21.1 percent to approximately 18.3 percent. That means for 100 women like Mary eating a Mediterranean Diet, only 18 of them would likely have a stroke over their lifetime.

TIP

It's important to recognize that when you hear about absolute risk reductions or increases, you often deal with relatively small numbers. Sometimes it seems disappointing or far less "shocking" than media headlines may have you believe.

Health trends: Prevalence and incidence data

Understanding prevalence and incidence is also crucial when discussing the impact of health conditions on a population. These two terms provide valuable insights into the frequency and occurrence of diseases within a specific group of people or geographical region.

Consider their definitions:

>> **Prevalence** refers to the total number of existing cases of a disease within a population at a given point in time. It provides a snapshot of how widespread the condition is within a particular group.

>> **Incidence,** on the other hand, measures the rate at which new cases or diagnoses of a disease develop within a population over a defined period, typically a year. It gives you an understanding of how quickly a disease spreads or pops up within the community.

Understanding Genetic Risk Factors and Family History

Genetic risk factors and family history are pivotal in shaping your risk or susceptibility to certain brain health diseases. Like weights on the scales, genetic predispositions often tip the balance toward specific health issues.

Example: Huntington's disease and genetic risk factors

One poignant example of the impact of genetic predisposition is Huntington's disease (HD). HD is a severe neurological condition caused by a faulty gene on chromosome 4, which produces the huntington protein. The disease is dominantly inherited, meaning each child of an affected parent has a 50 percent chance of inheriting the gene. This risk is independent for each child, like flipping a coin, and affects males and females equally.

Example: Alzheimer's disease and genetic risk factors

When considering Alzheimer's disease (AD), the role of genetic risk factors is more complicated. AD involves more complex genetic factors, with no single gene causing it. However, the APOE ε4 allele on chromosome 19 increases the risk of developing AD. About 14 percent of people carry this allele, but even those with two copies don't always develop AD, showing the complex relationship between genes and environment in this disease.

Nurturing Brain Health through Lifestyle Choices

Like weights on the scale, the various choices you make during your lifetime can tip the balance toward different outcomes, ranging from optimal brain function to the onset of neurodegenerative diseases.

REMEMBER

While genetic predispositions may hold weight for some diseases, you hold a remarkable degree of agency over the factors influencing your brain health. Unlike your genes, which you can't tweak or change, lifestyle choices offer a tangible avenue for intervention — a chance to tip the scales in favor of cognitive vitality.

Lifestyle factors encompass all sorts of choices you make in your day-to-day life to shape the health and function of your brain. These factors go far beyond genetics and include concepts such as staying active, eating well, staying socially connected, challenging the mind, getting good sleep, managing stress, and being mindful of environmental influences. While some of these factors may seem a bit mundane or even inconsequential, they can quickly add up to exert a profound effect over time. By understanding and addressing what are known as *modifiable risk factors*, you can actively promote brain resilience and reduce your risk of cognitive decline.

Taking a Holistic View of Brain Health

Taking a big picture or holistic view of brain health and disease involves considering the intricate interplay of biological, psychological, and social factors in shaping cognitive function and well-being. By considering the big picture, you recognize that brain health is influenced by different factors, or "voices." Rather like a crowd of people, many voices are competing for attention. Sometimes one voice may be louder than the rest, while others may fade into the background (or we may pay attention to the wrong voice by mistake). However, all the voices add to the cognitive "choir."

The bio-psycho-social model, created in the late 20th century, led to a transformation in how to think about health and disease. It went beyond the biomedical model, which only looked at biological causes for poor health. The basic idea set out by the model is that health, human behavior, and mental processes disease are caused by the interaction of biological, psychological, and social factors.

The biopsychosocial model is a comprehensive framework for understanding the intricate interplay of biological, psychological, and social factors shaping human health and well-being. However, in grappling with the complexities of brain health, I developed a complementary model — The Bottom-Up, Outside-In, Top-Down framework — which places the brain at the center. (See Chapter 1 for more info on this model.) Drawing inspiration from the biopsychosocial model, this framework expands the scope of social factors to encompass interpersonal relationships and the broader environmental influences that permeate our senses. Not only do these many elements regulate the brain's development, performance, and health, but each element interacts with and influences others in dynamic ways.

2

Charting Brain Health at Different Ages and Stages

Learn how childhood experiences, maternal health, and relationships shape healthy brain development.

Understand the teenage brain's unique challenges, from puberty to mental health and social connections.

Explore how lifestyle choices impact brain aging, memory, and the risks of dementia.

Discover how sex and gender differences influence brain health, from hormones to unique risks for men and women.

Recognize the signs of brain injuries and understand their long-term effects on health and well-being.

Learn how your environment, from air quality to sunlight to urban living, impacts brain health.

IN THIS CHAPTER

» **Shaping brain development during critical periods**

» **Looking at maternal health and the first 1000 days**

» **Recognizing the importance of warm responsive relationships**

» **Understanding the impact of early trauma and toxic stress**

» **Educating through language and play**

Chapter **6**

Nurturing Healthy Brain Development in Childhood

Parenting: The role that comes with a lifetime contract. Speaking from the trenches of parenting teenagers, I can vouch for the trials, new quests, and battles that show up at every stage. I also know that laying a solid foundation during infancy and early childhood is like pouring the concrete for what will become a grand skyscraper. Now, as I'm busy navigating the challenges of parenting teenagers, I'm beginning to see the glimmers of that foundational work paying off.

Even if you haven't signed up for a "parenting position" yourself, this chapter is a look at what is required to successfully build a little person's brain. Whether you're raising a mini-you, or simply want to appreciate architectural plans, scaffolding, and neuro-building blocks, this chapter shows you what goes into constructing a healthy, happy brain.

From Chromosomes to Complexity

As early as two weeks after conception, even before a mom may realize she's pregnant, her embryo's nervous system is beginning to take shape. The nervous system is among the first organ system to start developing and among the last to finish — human brains continue to mature well into the late teenage years.

REMEMBER

Brain development starts when your father's sperm meets your mother's egg, setting your genetic blueprint. Females inherit two X chromosomes, one from each parent, while males inherit an X from their mother and a Y from their father. These 23 chromosome pairs hold DNA, containing the instructions for building a human.

Surprisingly, only about 20,000 genes make up this guide, with one-third coding for proteins in the nervous system. Despite 86 billion neurons and up to 100 trillion synapses, the limited number of genes underscores the brain's remarkable capacity for experience-dependent plasticity.

Building the brain: In utero

By the time a pregnancy is confirmed, the nervous system is already forming. After fertilization, the egg divides into a blastocyst, a hollow ball of cells that develops into the embryo. The brain and spinal cord emerge from the neural plate, which folds and closes to form the neural tube. Proper neural tube closure is critical to prevent birth defects like spina bifida. Folic acid is often recommended to help with this process, although the exact mechanism remains unclear.

The brain's 86 billion neurons begin as stem cells, which can divide endlessly and become any cell type. Neural stem cells generate all the brain's cells through neurogenesis, which is key to building the nervous system.

Around month five of pregnancy, neurogenesis peaks, but about half of the neurons die through *apoptosis*. This "cell suicide" helps regulate the number of neurons, ensuring the right balance, with nerve growth factors like BDNF playing a role in determining which neurons survive.

After neurons are born, they migrate to their final positions in the brain. They then grow dendrites and axons, which use growth cones to navigate and form connections with target neurons. This leads to *synaptogenesis*, the process of creating synaptic connections.

NEUROGENESIS IN ADULTS

The first description of adult human neurogenesis came from a landmark 1998 paper titled "Neurogenesis in the Adult Human Hippocampus" published in *Nature Medicine*. The research cleverly used carbon-14, a byproduct of Cold War nuclear tests, to date newly formed neurons. Carbon-14 is absorbed by plants and enters our DNA when we eat them, providing a timestamp for dividing cells. The study found that about 700 new neurons are added to each side of the human hippocampus daily. While this finding is promising for therapies, it represents only 0.004 percent of the total hippocampal neuron population, much lower than levels seen in lab animals.

The developing brain creates more synapses than it needs, but this surplus is pruned during infancy and childhood. Early on, pruning is guided by spontaneous neural activity, but later, it depends on sensory experiences, which shape the brain to fit its environment.

Building the brain: Infancy and childhood

As a newborn enters the world, their brain is roughly one-third the size of an adult brain, capable only of basic reflexes such as suckling, crying, and sleeping. However, from birth onward, the brain undergoes rapid growth and refinement through interactions with the environment.

Newborn reflexes

Reflexes are the automatic muscle responses that newborn babies show in response to certain types of stimulation. A pediatrician once said to me that reflexes are the secret handshakes of babyhood.

The top seven newborn reflexes are listed here:

>> **Rooting reflex:** Stroking the baby's cheek or mouth causes them to turn their head and search around for a nipple.

>> **Sucking reflex:** Compels the baby to suck when something touches their mouth.

>> **Moro reflex (startle reflex):** Triggered by a sudden movement or noise, this reflex causes the baby to throw their arms outward as if in fright.

>> **Tonic neck reflex (fencing posture):** When the baby's head turns to one side while lying on their back, the limbs on that side straighten out, resembling a fencer's stance.

>> **Stepping reflex:** If you hold a baby upright with their feet touching a flat surface, they'll make little stepping movements.

>> **Babinski reflex:** Stroking the sole of the foot causes the big toe to move upward and the other toes to fan out.

>> **Grasping reflex:** Touching the palm of the baby's hand or the bottom of their foot causes the baby to grasp tightly with their hand or curl their toes.

These newborn reflexes generally fade as the baby's brain matures, usually around four to six months as voluntary movements take over.

Developmental milestones

Within just two years, babies go from lifting their heads to running and climbing! They lose their early reflexes, master grabbing toys, and even start drawing. As they learn to understand commands and express themselves, their unique personalities start to shine. By school age, they're making friends, telling stories, creating art, and ready to take on the world.

Tables 6-1 and 6-2 chart expected developmental milestones and serve as a very rough guide for observing and supporting the typical progression of skills.

TABLE 6-1

Developmental Milestones from Birth to 12 Months

	Birth–3 Months	3–6 Months	6–12 Months
Social	Social smile. Reacts to sight of bottle or breast.	Laughs out loud. Responds to name: turns and looks.	Plays social games, such as "peek-a-boo," "pat-a-cake." Pushes things away they don't want.
Self-Help	Comforts self with thumb or pacifier.	Feeds self cracker.	Feeds self with spoon. Lifts cup to mouth and drinks.
Gross Motor/ Reflexes	Lifts head and chest when lying on tummy.	Sits alone, steady and without support.	Crawls around on hands and knees.
Fine Motor	Looks at and reaches for faces and toys.	Uses two hands to pick up large objects.	Picks up small objects (thumb and finger grasp).
Language	Cries in such a way parents can distinguish different types of needs. Makes sounds such as "uh."	Babbles, such as "da-da," "ma-ma," "ba-ba."	Understands phrases such as "No-no" and "All gone."

TABLE 6-2

Developmental Milestones from 12 Months to Five Years

	12-24 Months	2-3 Years	3-4 Years	4-5 Years
Social	Usually responds to correction - stops. Shows sympathy to others.	Plays games such as tag, hide and seek. Plays a role in "pretend" games.	Cooperates without supervision and conflict. Directs other kids.	Follows simple rules in board or card games.
Self-Help	Takes off open coat or shirt without help.	Dresses self with help. Washes and dries hands.	Dresses and undresses without help, except tying shoelaces.	Usually looks both ways before crossing road.
Gross Motor	Walks up and down stairs alone.	Rides around on tricycle, using pedals.	Hops on one foot without support.	Skips and jumps.
Fine Motor	Scribbles with crayon.	Cuts with small scissors.	Draws or copies a complete circle.	Draws a person with head, eyes, nose, mouth.
Language	Follows two-part instructions.	Answers questions. (For example, "Where do you put a hat?")	Talks in simple, complete sentences (ten+ words).	Reads a few letters (five+).

In terms of meeting milestones, parents and caregivers are often the first to sense something may be amiss. Regular healthy child check-ups and those all-important childhood vaccinations are not only crucial for keeping kids well, they provide opportunities for professionals to notice subtle nuances in your little one's development.

Brain development: Back to front

Brain development occurs sequentially, with different regions maturing at different stages. There's a sort of hierarchy of development starting with the basic sensory areas such as those for vision and touch and moving toward the cortical areas involved with complex thought. Rather than getting you bogged down in the age at which the visual cortex, thalamus, or hippocampus is predicted to mature, you may find it helpful to visualize this process by envisioning the brain developing from the inside out, then from the back to the front.

>> **Deeper subcortical regions (inside):** These regions, responsible for vital functions and basic reflexes such as suckling and grasping, reach maturity before the (outer) cortex.

>> **Primary sensory areas (back):** The primary sensory areas, such as those for vision, touch, and hearing, located in the occipital, parietal, and posterior temporal lobes respectively, mature early on.

>> **Language centers (middle):** Language centers in the temporal lobe then develop during infancy and early childhood. This middle-stage development emphasizes the importance of language acquisition and communication skills.

>> **Frontal lobes (front):** The frontal lobes, governing higher cognitive functions such as reasoning, planning, and emotion regulation, fully mature during adolescence and early adulthood.

REMEMBER

The process of brain development is orderly, follows a predictable pattern, and tracks alongside the emergence of well-established childhood language, social, and behavioral milestones. As brains get more organized, efficient, and sophisticated, so do the little owners of those brains!

Shaping the Developing Brain: Critical Periods for Brain Development

Throughout infancy, childhood, and adolescence, all life experiences — whether nurturing or challenging — imprint themselves on the developing brain. The experiences a child has become even more pronounced during critical periods of neurodevelopment — windows of time when the brain is especially sensitive to specific environmental stimuli, which can shape, enhance, or impede the maturation process in profound and enduring ways.

What are critical periods?

Critical periods (sometimes called sensitive periods) are very specific windows of time and opportunity when the brain not only uses but often *requires* very specific sensory experiences to shape brain architecture.

REMEMBER

When these special windows of opportunity are open, the brain is especially plastic or changeable. Outside of these critical periods or after the windows close, the brain is less plastic or changeable, making it more challenging to develop new skills or hit milestones. Critical period timing follows a similar pattern to how the brain develops "back to front." Infant brains, for example, rapidly develop abilities such as vision, language, and social skills during cortical crucial periods. As you can see in Figure 6-1, critical periods for the primary senses of vision, hearing, and touch occur first, followed by language and, finally, higher order cognitive skills. The sequential opening and shutting of key periods mirrors the course of structural brain development.

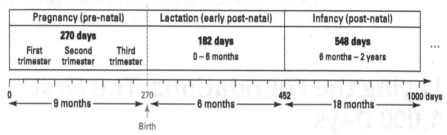

Pregnancy (pre-natal)			Lactation (early post-natal)	Infancy (post-natal)	
270 days			**182 days**	**548 days**	...
First trimester	Second trimester	Third trimester	0 – 6 months	6 months – 2 years	

FIGURE 6-1: Critical periods of child development.

0 ◄——— 9 months ———► 270 ◄——— 6 months ———► 452 ◄——— 18 months ———► 1000 days

Birth

© John Wiley & Sons, Inc.

REMEMBER

Experience can still modify adult brains, but it takes more effort because most critical periods have closed. Adults who have tried to learn a second language for the first time know that it's not impossible to become fluent, but it's never as easy as in childhood when the window for learning language is flung wide open. In adulthood, you can learn new skills, but the changes are subtler and tougher to acquire.

TIP

You may find it useful to think of the brain's activity and plasticity as resembling the scene inside a concert hall before the performance begins. Before the onset of a critical period, it's comparable to the audience's background chatter and the orchestra warming up. As the critical period commences, it's as though the conductor steps onto the podium, baton in hand, bringing order to the chaos. With the conductor's first gesture, the audience quiets and the orchestra starts to play in harmony.

Why are critical periods so critical?

During critical periods, every event or sensory experience has a consequential impact on brain wiring. But it's not just the stimuli that a baby or toddler experiences that matters; the *absence* of expected stimuli can have a profoundly detrimental effect. Two examples highlight this: the role of language and vision during early development.

>> **Hearing language:** Infants first understand and then speak words, a process that begins with babbling around three months. For deaf children, the first year is crucial. Without early hearing aids or cochlear implants, language and cognitive skills may suffer. However, deaf children exposed to sign language from birth learn naturally, avoiding many challenges faced by those without early intervention.

>> **Seeing:** Children born with strabismus (squint) need early correction to develop depth perception. Without treatment, like using an eye patch, they risk developing lazy eye (amblyopia), where the brain ignores input from one eye. Early intervention is essential, as the critical period for depth perception eventually closes, making correction much harder.

Laying the Foundations: The First 1,000 Days

As shown in Figure 6-2, there are roughly 1,000 days from conception until a child reaches their second birthday. These 1,000 days are formally recognized as a window of opportunity in which to build a healthy foundation for a child to grow, learn, and become a contributing member of their society in adulthood. I also calculated that if you count 10,000 days from conception, voila!, you'll have a teenager!

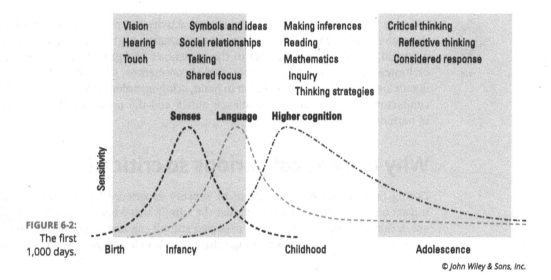

FIGURE 6-2: The first 1,000 days.

© John Wiley & Sons, Inc.

Maternal health matters

Recognizing this crucial first 1000-day period, global organizations such as the World Health Organization, the United Nations, and numerous government health agencies now emphasize the importance of promoting child health started from conception. The First 1000 Days programs advocate for the health of the child and also their mother, highlighting how it's important to treat pregnant and breast-feeding women as whole people, supporting and tending to their physical, mental, and social needs, too. By putting the health of mothers first and giving them full support during pregnancy and the first few years of life, a child's healthy growth is also supported.

Here are some take-aways from the first 1000 days maternal health priorities. These priorities have been designed to address the importance of diet and nutrition, maternal stress and trauma, avoiding toxins and infections, and maternal healthcare:

>> Maternal diet affects infant immunity and brain development; prioritize a healthy balance of fruits, vegetables, proteins, and whole grains (and avoid junk food!). Also, avoid the effects of undernutrition (malnutrition) on infant growth and the dangers of chronic disease caused by overnutrition (that is, processed foods).

>> Manage maternal stress to protect fetal development; minimize trauma and stress where possible.

>> Avoid alcohol, tobacco, and toxins to safeguard brain development.

>> Avoid and prevent infectious disease and other illnesses with good hygiene, vaccinations, and minimizing exposure to unwell people.

>> Prioritize early pregnancy detection and regular prenatal care to optimize early developmental outcomes.

TIP

You may notice I don't mention much here about the importance of infant and childhood sleep. Instead, sleep is covered in detail in Chapter 14.

Childhood nutrition and growth

It's important to ensure the unborn baby and the infant once born, get adequate nutrition at every stage. WHO and United Nations International Children's Emergency Fund (UNICEF) established the Global Strategy for Infant and Young Child Feeding as a response to the imperative of fostering growth, health, and survival in children, beginning with robust maternal nutrition.

Here's a summary for moms-to-be, or mothers who are breastfeeding and those helping prepare family meals:

>> **Pregnancy:** Eat a well-balanced diet with essential nutrients for baby's development.

- » **Breastfeeding:** Offer exclusive breast milk for the first six months for optimal nutrition and immunity. If breastfeeding directly isn't possible, expressing breast milk to be fed by bottle can be a helpful alternative, ensuring the baby still receives the benefits of breast milk.

- » **Introducing solids:** Begin with simple foods at six months and gradually diversify, avoiding added salt and sugar.

- » **Transition to family diet:** From about 12 months, shift to the family diet, ensuring proper intake of protein, vitamins, and minerals.

REMEMBER

Breastfeeding offers the ideal nutrition for infants as it equips them with all the essential nutrients they need from a healthy mother's milk. Also, the act of breastfeeding fosters crucial mom-baby attachment and emotional well-being. However, some moms face challenges that make breastfeeding difficult or impossible. In such cases, I feel that the statement, "breast is best" should be followed by a pragmatic ". . .but not at all costs." A fed, nourished, and well-loved baby should be the priority. Thankfully, formula feeding offers a valuable alternative to many families, providing essential nutrients for infant health when breastfeeding isn't working out.

The Importance of Warm, Caring Relationships

In this section, you discover why a solid, dependable bond with a caring adult can be a game-changer for kids, fostering resilience, and a hearty dose of lifelong good health. It turns out, adults are super important for providing the necessary emotional and cognitive toolkit to help little people learn to cope with life's ups and downs.

Building secure connections

Therapists, researchers in the social sciences, and healthcare professionals from psychology to psychiatry have long deliberated over why some people manage to navigate their traumatic childhoods successfully while others struggle as adults. Despite the diverse sources of stress or trauma — poverty, parental addiction or mental illness, warfare, violence, neglect, or a mix of these factors — the common denominator for those children who do well seems to be presence of at least one consistent, supportive loving bond with an adult such as a parent or caregiver.

Attachment theory 101

Attachment theory is a psychological model that suggests the bonds formed between children and their primary caregivers (usually this is their mom) are fundamental to how they form relationships later in life. British psychiatrist John Bowlby developed the model to explain how early attachment experiences influence a child's emotional, social, and cognitive growth. He argued that a secure attachment to a caregiver provides a child with a sense of safety and security that is essential for exploration and learning.

In an attached infant-parent/caregiver relationship four key attributes are observed.

>> **Safe haven.** Ideally, an attached youngster can seek solace from their parent or caregiver if they feel threatened, afraid, or in danger.

>> **Secure base.** Here, the parent or caregiver provides a solid and dependable foundation for the child to build on while they learn and solve problems on their own.

>> **Proximity maintenance.** This signifies that the child wants to explore the world but also wants to be close to his caregiver. For example, a toddler may play with toys at playgroup but regularly bring the toys back to show their mom.

>> **Separation distress.** This means that the child becomes unhappy and cries and sad when they're left behind or taken from their parent or caregiver.

According to Bowlby, the nature of attachment developed in childhood can persist into adulthood, shaping behavior in relationships, the ability to handle emotions, and stress. Securely attached individuals tend to have healthy relationships and a strong sense of self-worth, whereas those with insecure attachments may struggle with intimacy, trust, and self-esteem.

What do emotionally responsive relationships look like?

If you ever spend time with a baby, or watch parents interact with a newborn, you likely see them respond in a very particular way. Mother–infant synchrony (or any primary caregiver–infant interaction) is typically characterized by very touching face-to-face interactions including eye gaze, gentle touch, mimicking of facial expressions and emotions, and "motherese" or "baby talk."

"Motherese" now more inclusively known as "parentese" or "caretakerese," is the melodious, high-pitched way we naturally speak to infants. It captures their attention with its simplicity and rhythm. This form of speech, filled with elongated vowels and expressive tones, transcends languages and cultures. It's key for a baby's emotional engagement and linguistic development, often used by older children when interacting with younger ones as well.

Showing empathy and responsiveness

An environment in which parents or caregivers are perceptive and receptive to a young child's signals and needs literally shapes brain architecture. As the Harvard Center on the Developing Child states, "Because responsive relationships are both expected and essential, their absence is a serious threat to a child's development and well-being."

Even as young as a few months old, babies don't behave as passive "receivers" of attention. They start to demand it. Firstly, they use non-verbal cues (such as waving their arms or making eye contact) and later, as they get older, they start to use their words (including the inevitable "why" questions) and actions (bringing a toy over or pointing at objects such as trucks or animals).

Learning how to "serve and return"

The back and forward requests for attention and conversation are sometimes called "serve and return" interactions. Think of these as a game of tennis or ping pong where the baby "serves" a gesture or sound, and the caregiver "returns" with a response. This back-and-forth is not just fun; it's necessary for developing a sturdy brain architecture.

Here are five tips for parents learning how to "serve and return" to create responsive, warm attachments.

>> Notice the serve and share of the child's focus of attention. By noticing serves, you learn a lot about children's abilities, interests, and needs, and you can encourage them to explore.

>> Return the serve by supporting and encouraging. Make a sound or facial expression — such as saying, "I see!" or smiling and nodding to let a child know that you're noticing the same thing.

>> Name what a child is seeing, doing, or feeling, and you're making essential language connections in their brain.

>> Take turns . . . and then wait. Keep the interaction going back and forth.

>> Practice endings and beginnings. When you share a child's focus, you notice when they're ready to end the activity and begin something new.

WARNING

Unreliable, inappropriate, or nonexistent replies from adults to a child's requests for conversation, play, or attention can disturb the brain's developing architecture, resulting in physical, mental, and emotional health issues. Harvard Center on the Developing Child states that neglect is a "double whammy" because the child lacks the appropriate relational to-and-fro stimulation it expects, *and* it activates the child's stress response system needlessly.

Parenting well when you're worn out

If you're busy raising happy little children, you know it's not feasible to always be responding to your child 100 percent of the time. You won't be able to catch every "serve" your child bats your way. But please don't fret about causing irreversible harm to your child's brain wiring! You can miss a few serves, and still stay in the match.

TIP

Remember, parenting isn't about 100 percent constant responsiveness and "returning" every "serve," but about being "good enough" and providing safety and love.

Educating Little Brains

If you remember them, think back at your preschool or early school days. What details do you recall? My memories of my four-year-old Kindy are vivid and precious. I can still see the cloakroom's hooks marked with pictures, the playdoh cakes that were popular for fifth birthdays, and the hours spent pushing go-carts. You may remember painting, reading, playing with friends, or feeding the kindergarten fish. These aren't just nostalgic snapshots; they represent the foundation of essential life skills. Early childhood education plays a critical role in shaping cognitive and social abilities, setting the stage for lifelong learning and development.

Nurturing development of executive functions

Children are not born with mature executive function skills — they can't always control their emotions, make plans, stay focused, read or solve complex math problems. But they're born with the *potential* to develop these capabilities. So long as they're exposed to rich learning experiences.

Executive function skills help you to plan, focus attention, switch between tasks, and juggle multiple ideas at once. There are three core aspects to executive functioning skills. You may like to think how they may apply to yourself and to different ages of children:

>> Working memory lets you hold onto information and apply it as needed.

>> Inhibitory control helps you manage your thoughts and impulses, enabling you to resist distractions and act thoughtfully.

>> Cognitive flexibility enables you to adapt to new situations, shift priorities, and see concepts from different angles.

TIP

The Harvard Center on the Developing Child likens executive function skills to air traffic control at a busy airport. Think of executive function and self-regulation skills as an air traffic control system masterfully coordinating the coming and going of flights on multiple runways. These skills help little people learn and use information, focus, tune out distractions, and smoothly transition between tasks.

WARNING

Children who struggle with these skills early on may face academic challenges, have difficulty following directions, and experience issues forming positive relationships with peers.

Language development through talking, reading, and singing

Children learn and develop best through play. Children and other young mammals (speaking as a puppy owner!) are driven by a natural urge to explore, discover, touch, taste, and immerse themselves in their surroundings, including interactions with people and animals, or even the simple joy found in kitchen cupboards and the muddy puddles. This intense interaction with their environment is crucial for brain development, as little brains are wired to absorb and grow from experiences.

The Harvard Center on the Developing Child emphasizes the importance of engaging, age-appropriate games and activities to enhance different aspects of executive function in children.

Here are some fun ideas for age-appropriate play to promote executive skill development.

>> **Infants (6–18 months):** Lap games such as Peekaboo and Pat-a-Cake boost memory and self-control.

- **Toddlers (18 months–3 years):** Play Follow the Leader and engage in storytelling for cognitive growth.

- **Preschoolers (3–5 years):** Use structured imaginary play and group storytelling to develop complex thinking.

- **Early School Age (5–7 years):** Introduce games such as Go Fish to challenge memory and strategy skills.

- **Older Children (7–12 years):** Chess and music instruments (and dare I say online gaming!) hone mental flexibility and attention.

Navigating out-of-home childcare

The preschool years are some of the most important years of a little person's life and certainly when the foundations of language development, executive functioning, social and emotional development, self-regulation and problem-solving skills, are laid down.

Fostering a good childhood in ECEC

Early childhood education and care (ECEC), especially if its outside of the home, is an important decision many families agonize over. You may need to weigh your work and financial commitments with your desire for a safe and caring experience for your infant or toddler.

Access to high-quality ECEC is linked to improved social and cognitive skills, indicating its vital role in early development. However, studies into ECEC present a nuanced picture, with mixed outcomes that hinge on the nature of ECEC — ranging from government-run preschools to informal arrangements such as care by grandparents.

Notably, preschoolers between ages three and four who attend high-caliber ECEC programs generally demonstrate better academic and social readiness for school compared to those who don't. Numerous studies show the positive impacts of ECEC are especially for children from disadvantaged backgrounds, highlighting ECEC's role in providing equitable developmental opportunities. In their recommendation for early childcare, UNICEF states, "Quality pre-primary education is the foundation of a child's journey."

WARNING

Any discussion around children younger than three attending out-of-home ECEC is sensitive and complex. Research suggests that for children living in healthy nurturing homes, high-quality childcare before the age of three doesn't necessarily lead to better cognitive and language development. On the other hand, poor quality childcare may cause harm. For example, spending excessive time in group care from an early age may be linked to behavioral issues later. Central to a child's well-being is the availability of nurturing and responsive care, irrespective of whether it is provided at home or in a childcare facility.

Defining high-quality ECEC

What makes for high-quality childcare? Luckily, organizations such as UNICEF provide guidelines. As part of assessing the quality of ECEC, here are some questions to ask yourself:

>> Are caregivers providing warm, responsive interactions? And is the teacher-to-child ratio low enough for individual attention?

>> Is there a structured, fun educational framework? And does the environment offer affection, stability, and varied activities?

>> Can I be actively involved in the childcare experience?

>> Is the center culturally sensitive and inclusive?

Untangling the Impact of Early Childhood Trauma and Toxic Stress

When you feel scared, nervous, or excited, it's completely normal for your heart rate and blood pressure to rise, along with an increase in stress hormones such as cortisol. These changes prepare your body for action. Usually, these responses normalize again, settling down to a healthy calm baseline. The process of activating and then returning to a baseline state is the sign of a healthy robust stress response system.

The stress-response system goes through its own sensitive period of development during infancy and early childhood. When young children are nurtured within a loving and supportive family environment free from trauma, they develop healthy robust stress response systems. However, if children are exposed to excessive or toxic stress in the absence of caring, protective relationships, they may be unable to develop adequate stress responses. Early life stress has long-lasting and extensive impacts.

Defining different types of stress

Because not all stress is bad, language has evolved to describe three distinct types of stress each affecting children differently and requiring different levels of support and intervention.

» **Positive stress** (sometimes called eustress) is an expected part of everyday life and includes manageable challenges that, with the right support, help children grow and learn resilience. Think of a child feeling nervous about their first day at a new school. It's a situation that may make them feel uneasy, but with encouragement and support from their family, they can face the challenge, make new friends, and come out stronger for it.

» **Tolerable stress** (sometimes called distress) involves more significant events that could disrupt a child's development but are manageable with strong, supportive relationships. Imagine a child who experiences the loss of a grandparent. This loss is a big challenge for a little person, but with love and support from their family, they can navigate through their grief, understanding and accepting their emotions in a healthy way.

» **Toxic stress** (sometimes called trauma) is the kind of stress that can cause lasting harm to a child's health and development. This involves intense and ongoing challenges without adequate adult support, such as living in a home with constant conflict or neglect or extreme poverty. In such cases, the child's stress response is activated so often that it can affect their brain health and development, making it harder for them to manage stress appropriately in the future.

Toxic stress: A huge disrupter of brain development

As you discover earlier in this chapter, the brain is rapidly developing during early childhood, making it highly plastic — it's adapting, growing, and changing more during this period than at any other time in life. Critical periods are when the brain is very responsive to learning by experience, an upside of brain plasticity. However, the flip side is during critical periods of development that young brains are also very vulnerable to negative influences, including toxic stress or trauma.

WARNING

When a child experiences toxic stress, it can disrupt the brain's development. Given that critical periods are windows of plasticity *and* vulnerability to stress, you can see why toxic stress in early childhood is particularly damaging.

It's not only the brain undergoing rapid development during infancy and early childhood, but the stress-response system is also learning how to react to the world. When infants or children experience toxic stress, their stress-response system is over-activated so often it learns the world is dangerous. This leads to children overreacting to situations that aren't threatening or remaining hyper-vigilant or anxious long after the stressful experience is over. In short, it's harder to cope with adversity and become resilient.

Adverse childhood experiences (ACES)

Adverse Childhood Experiences (ACEs), describe various forms of toxic stress a child may experience growing up. ACEs were first identified in a pivotal study by the Centers for Disease Control (CDC) and Kaiser Permanente in 1995. This research found ACEs are surprisingly common with around two in three people reporting at least one ACE, and a notable percentage experiencing three or more.

What are ACEs?

As the number of ACEs increases, so does the risk for negative health outcomes later in life. For example, people with lots of ACES are at higher risk for metabolic disease, heart disease, mental health issues, and socioeconomic struggles. However, there isn't a specific threshold number of ACEs that will guarantee poor health in adulthood.

Here is a list of ACEs as first described by the CDC:

>> **Physical neglect:** Failure to supervise or provide for the child

>> **Emotional neglect:** Caregiver unable to express affection or love for the child due to personal problems

>> **Physical abuse:** Severe assault or physical abuse such as shaking or hitting

>> **Sexual abuse:** Child experiences sexual abuse or forced sex

>> **Emotional abuse:** Caregiver engaged in psychological aggression toward the child such as threatening

>> **Caregiver treated violently:** Domestic violence of an adult in the home including slapping hitting or kicking

>> **Caregiver substance abuse:** Active alcohol and drug abuse by a caregiver

>> **Caregiver mental illness:** Serious mental illness or elevated mental health symptoms

>> **Caregiver divorce/family separation:** Child's parent(s) deceased, separated, or divorced or child is abandoned or placed in out-of-home care

>> **Caregiver incarceration:** Caregiver spent time in prison or is currently in jail or detention center

The original ACEs study focused on personal and family hardship, but the list has since expanded to include broader community and socio-economic issues such as violence, discrimination, and poverty, recognizing that the stress response system reacts to threats from any source, not just within the home.

WARNING

It's important to recognize that although there's a correlation between ACEs and poorer health outcomes in adulthood, this isn't a universal rule that applies to every person. Individual experiences and outcomes can differ significantly. Not everyone with ACEs is guaranteed poor adult health, highlighting the resilience and unique paths of healing that people can find.

Mitigating the effects of ACES with early intervention

To shield children from the harms of toxic stress, one key strategy stands out: nurturing strong, warm relationships with caring adults. These bonds provide children with stability and affection, help them learn to manage their behavior, and foster essential life skills. This nurturing presence acts as a shield or buffer, offering children a safe haven or secure base that helps them face challenges and grow stronger.

Creating an environment that cultivates resilience involves several protective factors, known as PACES — protective factors for adverse childhood experiences. Ten PACES have been identified that fall into two categories: supportive relationships and enriching resources.

Supportive relationship PACES include:

>> Receiving unconditional love from a caregiver

>> Having a best friend to confide in

>> Engaging in community service as a volunteer

>> Being an active member of a group or club

>> Benefiting from the guidance of a mentor

Enriching resources PACEs contribute to a child's learning, stress management, and avoiding risky behaviors. These resources are:

>> Living in a secure and safe home environment

>> Accessing quality education opportunities

>> Enjoying hobbies and leisure activities

>> Participating in regular physical activity

>> Following established household rules and routines

TIP

The good news is that it's never too late to foster resilience. Through healthy activities suited to their age, such as regular exercise, stress management, and skill-building programs, children and adults alike can improve their capacity to handle adversity. Adults can amplify this effect by embodying resilient behaviors themselves, thus setting a strong example for the younger generation. But governments and policymakers must also play a role in facilitating this process by supporting families. Essentially, it's about crafting a network of support to grow healthy children, especially those facing toxic stress: No one (and certainly never a child) should have to navigate challenges alone.

PLAYING IS FOR CHILDREN

The process of enjoyable learning and skill acquisition is heavily reliant on these experiences to enhance neural connections. Human brains, complex and socially oriented as they are, require a prolonged period of rich childhood experiences. It's been said an extended childhood enables brains to better match the rich experiences and diverse environments people inhabit around the world.

Encourage children to play! It's the key to sculpting a healthy, developing brain. Remember that children do not grow in a vacuum; their environments have a significant impact on their thoughts, emotions, and behaviors. Allow them to splash in puddles (children are washable!), make music with kitchenware, and get up close with nature. By creating a rich warm loving environment, you're not only developing their minds, but also assisting in the development of their distinct identities. So go ahead and promote the mess, noise, and adventure. Their little brains will thank you for it!

IN THIS CHAPTER

» Looking at the teenage brain

» Navigating the hormones of puberty

» Cultivating teenage social bonds and identity

» Understanding mental health in adolescence

» Assessing adolescents' risky behaviors

Chapter **7**

Fostering Healthy Brain Development in Adolescence

This chapter isn't just for those in the throes of raising a teenager or two (as I am as I write this book) — it's a chance to reflect for all of us. Whether you're actively shaping a young mind, struggling to keep a teen on the right tracks, or looking back on your formative years with a mix of nostalgia or relief, there's common ground in the universal journey of adolescence.

From a brain health perspective, the neural pathways of the teenage brain are highly plastic and easily shaped by experience, molding lifelong patterns of behavior, mood, and memories. Here, I explore the elements that contribute to a teenager's brain development and good health, including the resilience and vulnerability unique to this critical period.

Adolescence: A Sensitive Phase of Brain Development

Adolescence is usually defined as the phase of life between childhood and adulthood. It involves significant changes to the body, brain, and the way a young person interacts with the world. Among neuroscientists, adolescence is now recognized as another critical (although usually now they use the term "sensitive") period of brain development.

Adolescence is a period of profound social, psychological, and biological change. Here are some of the main changes taking place:

>> With the onset of puberty, boys' and girls' bodies change rapidly, and hormones such as estrogen and testosterone (T) surge, affecting everything from mood to metabolism.

>> Friendships take center stage as teens start to prioritize friends over family, with friendships shaping their social skills and identity.

>> Some teens find themselves on an emotional rollercoaster of heightened sensitivity and mood swings.

>> The teenage brain enters a sensitive period of development and shows extensive grey and white matter reorganization and network development.

>> Adolescents become drawn to new experiences and risks, driven by brain circuits related to reward processing. The end goal here is independence, which takes courage and a dose of bravado.

>> Teens begin to explore their own values and beliefs, striving for autonomy and self-reliance.

Tracking the beginning and end of adolescence

The onset of puberty is commonly considered the beginning of adolescence. However, no clear biological indicator signifies the end of this stage.

Although the societal end point of adolescence may be fuzzy, its biological importance is crystal clear: This stage is as critical for brain development as infancy and childhood. Driven by sex hormones, the adolescent brain becomes plastic again, and it's a time when the brain's cognitive, emotional, and social neural networks undergo streamlining and fine-tuning. Interestingly, many of the typical behavioral shifts you may see in teenagers are a direct reflection of these developmental changes in the brain.

Charting adolescent brain development

Child and adolescent brain researchers mostly agree on several key points about young people's brain development:

>> Early childhood is marked by an increase in cortical grey matter volume, which peaks in late childhood. Throughout adolescence, the frontal, parietal, and temporal cortices experience a reduction in both volume and thickness, a process that stabilizes in the early twenties.

>> White matter increases in volume and organization into adulthood, peaking at around age 30. Recall that white matter is white because of myelin which insulates axons, thus accelerating signaling between different brain regions.

>> Not all parts of the brain mature at the same rate during adolescence. For example, the gray matter volume of the caudate, putamen, and nucleus accumbens decreases with age, whereas the volume trajectories of the amygdala, cerebellum, hippocampus, pallidum, and thalamus display an inverted U-shaped pattern (that is, they expand slightly, then shrink again).

>> Sex differences in the trajectory of brain development emerge during adolescence. Typically, girls achieve their maximum grey matter volume (cortical and subcortical) a bit earlier than boys. But this variation is influenced mainly by the onset of puberty, which, on average, begins for girls about a year earlier than for boys. So, boys eventually catch up.

Minding the gap: The developmental mismatch model

One popular idea in neuroscience concerning adolescent brain development is the "mismatch theory." The theory suggests that undesirable teenage behaviors such as risk-taking, emotional instability, and self-absorption stem from uneven maturation between subcortical regions, which handle emotional reactions and risk versus reward processing, and the prefrontal cortex (PFC), responsible for cognitive control.

This theory claims the PFC doesn't fully mature until age 25. While there's evidence supporting different brain structures maturing at different rates, critics argue the age-25 cut-off is arbitrary and misleading. They question the labeling of younger brains as "immature" and note that this mismatch doesn't always correlate with the typical adolescent behaviors we see.

Losing grey matter: Less is sometimes more!

REMEMBER

Losing grey matter during adolescence (or any time of life) may sound bad, but in the teenage brain's case, this isn't a loss; it's a smart move! The brain keeps the connections that are important — the ones being used — and gets rid of the rest. This process embodies the principle of "use it or lose it."

Now, get out your trusty microscope as you're going to peer more closely at the grey matter to see what is happening at the cellular level. During childhood, the brain's grey matter, which is made up of neuron cell bodies, dendrites, and unmyelinated axons thickens as it adds new neurons and glia and creates neural connections, or synapses. As it enters adolescence, there's a shift: The brain begins to refine, prune, and tune these connections. As you can see in Figure 7-1, before puberty, the density of the dendritic spines in children is three times higher than in early adulthood. The pruning of unwanted connections adds up to volume loss and "thinning" of the cortex.

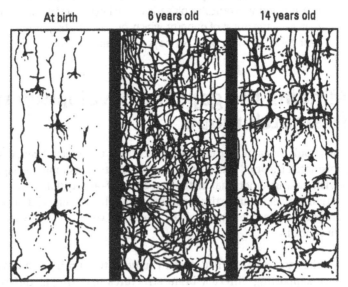

Synaptic Density

At birth   6 years old   14 years old

© John Wiley & Sons, Inc.

FIGURE 7-1:
Changes in synapse density from childhood to adolescence.

Grey matter volume changes follow a back-to-front wave, with sensory and motor areas maturing first and higher-order regions like the PFC, responsible for executive function and decision-making, and regions such as the temporal and parietal lobes, which handle social cognition, maturing last.

Adolescence is critical — period!

In neuroscience, its understood that the human brain is incredibly responsive to experiences — especially during early childhood and adolescence. This capacity is referred to as *experience-dependent plasticity*. As I mention in Chapter 6, *critical periods* are times when experiences and biological factors come together to significantly shape how the brain's circuits are wired.

Adolescence is now widely recognized as the critical period for the maturation of executive functions, including behavioral and cognitive abilities and social cognition. This phase is crucial for refining skills that govern decision-making, self-regulation, and social interactions.

Halcyon days: The reminiscence bump of adolescence

TIP

If you're over 40, here's a fun example illustrating that adolescence is indeed a highly sensitive period for brain development. The term "reminiscence bump" refers to the vivid autobiographical memories you have of ages 13 to 30. As a Gen Xer, my peers and I are hitting 50, so we're celebrating with nostalgic 90s-themed parties featuring double-denim, "Rachel" haircuts, and the era's hits from the Spice Girls, Oasis, and Nirvana.

You form identities and social bonds through shared cultural experiences such as music and movies during your young adult years. The strength of your reminiscing is due to several key factors: your plastic adolescent brain, the novelty of first-time experiences, their significant role in shaping your life and identity, and the personal and professional decisions you made as you started to take control of your own life.

Navigating Puberty

Every child follows their own individual pathway through puberty — some are early bloomers, others are late-starters. But puberty isn't only about the physical changes. It involves the beginning of neurodevelopmental, emotional, and behavioral changes unlike any seen since infancy.

Tracking the changes of puberty

Around age eight, children experience adrenarche, an early puberty stage where the adrenal glands start producing hormones. These hormones eventually lead to changes such as the growth of pubic and underarm hair, adult body odor, and acne (all the fun stuff!). Although these hormones, including androgens such as T and its precursor dehydroepiandrosterone (DHEA), are often thought of as "male" hormones, they're important for both boys and girls.

From a strictly evolutionary perspective, puberty is all about getting the body and brain ready to date, mate, and nurture offspring. In both boys and girls, it begins with the activation of the hypothalamic-pituitary-gonadal (HPG) axis, which results in:

>> Maturation of gametes (oocytes/eggs in the ovaries of girls, spermatozoa in the testes of boys)

>> Increased levels of sex hormones (ovarian hormones in girls; testicular hormones in boys), and adrenal hormones (in both boys and girls)

>> Appearance of secondary sex characteristics (body hair, breasts and such in girls, larger penis, testicles, and muscles in boys)

>> Fertility (menstrual cycle in girls and ability to ejaculate in boys)

REMEMBER

Puberty results in the maturation of a body capable of reproduction, while adolescence sharpens the social, emotional, and cognitive skills needed for it; however, it's often best to wait for parenthood until both the mind and life circumstances align, providing more opportunities for potential parents and their future families.

A primer on pubertal hormones

During puberty, the HPG axis plays a crucial role in initiating and regulating the hormonal changes that occur in the body. This axis involves a complex set of feedback mechanisms between the hypothalamus (which produces gonadotropin-releasing hormone; GnRH), the pituitary gland (which releases luteinizing hormone; LH and follicle-stimulating hormone; FSH), and the gonads (which produce sex steroids).

Puberty begins with KISS

A gene known as KISS-1, located in a small group of neurons within the hypothalamus, regulates the release of GnRH. KISS-1 codes for a protein known as kisspeptin. *Kisspeptin* acts on GnRH neurons in the hypothalamus to kick-start the process of puberty. During childhood, there is a tiny amount of GnRH released, but instead of an adult-like rhythmic tick-tick-tick, release is low, slow, and continuous. This low-level steady release effectively silences the entire HPG axis resulting in a sort of "hormonal hibernation" (or less technically, childhood) a phase of life unique to humans and a few higher order primates.

Alongside kisspeptin, the neurons release two additional peptide hormones, neurokinin B and dynorphin, collectively known as KNDy, which sounds like "candy." The origins of these names have an interesting backstory. KISS-1 was identified by researchers at the Pennsylvania State University College of Medicine in Hershey. This gene was named KISS-1 as a tribute to the Hershey's kisses, named after the local chocolate factory.

The hormones of puberty

Here are the hormones that begin to be released at puberty in both boys and girls:

- **Gonadotropin-releasing Hormone (GnRH):** Released by the hypothalamus GnRH stimulates the pituitary gland to release LH and FSH.

- **Luteinizing Hormone (LH):** Released by the pituitary gland LH stimulates the gonads (ovaries or testes) to produce sex hormones.

- **Follicle-stimulating Hormone (FSH):** Also released by the pituitary gland FSH works with LH to facilitate gamete (eggs or sperm) production.

- **Testosterone (T; in boys):** Produced by the testes, T drives the development of male secondary sexual characteristics, such as increased muscle mass, voice deepening, and growth of body hair.

- **Estrogen (in girls):** Produced by the ovaries, estrogen leads to the development of female secondary sexual characteristics, such as breast growth, menstrual cycle initiation, and body shape changes.

- **Progesterone (in girls):** Also produced by the ovaries, progesterone prepares the body for potential pregnancy post-ovulation, contributes to the regulation of the menstrual cycle.

These puberty-related hormones contribute to brain development and to promote sex differences in neural circuits. Thus, it stands to reason that changes in the way the brain works during puberty would show distinct trends in how girls and boys develop.

Sex hormones and brain reorganization

Your brain has receptors that recognize sex hormones, much like it does with neurotransmitters. When a hormone "key" fits into a receptor "lock", it turns on biological reactions in the cell. Sex hormone receptors, such as those for estrogen and testosterone, are found throughout the brain and influence how neurons communicate.

Sex hormones and brain organization in utero

There are two life phases when the brain is super sensitive to influence by sex hormones: in utero and during puberty. Neuroendocrinologists refer to these as the organization and activation phases.

>> **Organization:** During the initial sensitive phase in utero, sex hormones wire up or organize reproductive brain circuits.

>> **Activation:** The second sensitive phase is during puberty when sex hormones activate pre-organized reproductive brain circuits.

During the prenatal period, male fetal testes produce the dominating influence of T. T ensures reproductive regions of the brain in males become "masculinized." In females, in the absence of T, brain regions involved in reproductive behaviors in females become "feminized." Female sex hormones such as estrogen play no role — the developing female brain is thus a by-product of T's absence, rather than presence.

WARNING

I like to clarify that here, the terms "feminized" and "masculinized" refer specifically to the organization of reproductive brain circuitry and not to the current understanding of gender identity or expression.

MALE, FEMALE, OR MOSAIC?

You're probably keen to ask the curly question: How different are male and female brains? The most obvious physical differences emerge in brain size and the volume of certain regions, particularly at puberty. But in terms of function, men and women share a significant amount of cognitive and behavioral similarities, making it hard to guess someone's biological sex based on individual cognitive test scores. It's also challenging to separate the effects of biology — like genes and hormones — from environmental influences.

Neuroscientist Daphne Joel's concept of the "mosaic brain" suggests that brains are a blend of traits traditionally associated with either sex, along with neutral characteristics, highlighting the individuality and complexity of each person's brain.

Hormones during puberty and the developing adolescent brain

Because every person follows a different trajectory through puberty it makes sense to assume that brain development differs between people of the same age.

Research suggests that the stage of puberty, rather than chronological age, plays a more significant role in shaping adolescent brain development. The onset of puberty triggers key processes like grey matter pruning and white matter myelination, impacting how brain regions connect and communicate. It's thought that the surge in sex hormones during puberty opens a window of opportunity for the brain to be shaped by experiences, making this period critical for developing functions like executive control and social cognition. Without exposure to the appropriate cues—hormonal, educational, and social—the development of these key functions could face long-term consequences.

WARNING

If you're wondering about how puberty blockers used for children and young people with gender dysphoria affect the brain, the current evidence is scant in humans. A 2024 systematic review of the role of puberty suppression on brain development and cognition stated, "No human studies have systematically explored the impact of these treatments on neuropsychological function with an adequate baseline and follow up."

Understanding the impact of hormones on mood and behavior

REMEMBER

Blaming every bad mood a young person experiences on "hormones" is very easy. They're the obvious scapegoat (and this is especially the case for girls and women throughout their lifespan). But don't forget, puberty involves more than changing levels of sex hormones.

Teenagers are experiencing a multitude of changes including:

>> Fine tuning of neural networks and increased sensitivity of brain circuits that process emotions, social interactions, and new ways of thinking.

>> Shifts in relationships with parents, peers, and romantic partners, including exploring sexual identity, combined with increased social media use.

>> Developing their own sense of values and morals.

>> The transition from primary school to high school to decision-making about what to do upon graduation.

>> Growing awareness of the cultural and societal expectations of sex and gender and what this means to them personally.

That's not to say that teenagers aren't vulnerable to mood changes, mood disorders, or struggles with emotion regulation. But it's important to understand that mood changes are not solely caused by hormones. Later in the chapter, I explore the mental health vulnerabilities of adolescence in greater detail.

Cultivating Social Ties

It may seem obvious to point out that humans are inherently social, our survival and success are deeply rooted in the evolution of brain networks that support social behaviors. The "social brain" refers to the neural networks that equip you with the mental abilities to interpret social cues and act appropriately in social contexts. These skills include understanding and navigating complex social interactions, attracting partners, distinguishing friend from foe, and interpreting other people's emotions (empathy) and thoughts (mentalizing).

Describing the social brain

There's a tendency to think of the "social brain" in terms of cognition (or thinking) only. But there are three stages of social information processing:

>> **Social perception** is the innate or implicit phase where social cues such as smell, touch, facial recognition, and speech are perceived (that is, seen, heard, smelt, or felt).

>> **Social cognition** involves building an understanding of another human through social brain networks. Aspects include empathy, theory of mind, and rapid evaluations.

>> **Regulation and control of behavior** includes regulation of thoughts and actions in social contexts, including emotional recognition and social emotions.

Social brain neuroscientists interested in adolescent brain development focus on several key regions. These regions are part of a larger network that navigates increasingly complex social landscapes, identity formation, and emotion regulation. Social brain regions include:

>> **Prefrontal Cortex (PFC), Ventromedial Prefrontal Cortex (vMPFC), and Orbitofrontal Cortex (OFC):** Involved in processing rewards, guiding social behavior, and decision-making, especially in social contexts

>> **Amygdala:** Processing emotions and is linked to emotional and social learning

>> **Temporoparietal Junction (TPJ):** Engaged in theory of mind and empathy

>> **Superior Temporal Sulcus (STS):** Involved in perceiving where others are looking and interpreting facial expressions and body language

>> **Fusiform Face Area (FFA):** Specialized for facial recognition

>> **Anterior Cingulate Cortex (ACC):** Is important for error detection, social evaluation, and emotional response regulation

>> **Nucleus Accumbens (NAcc)/Vental Striatum:** Region associated with reward and pleasure, including social rewards

Social brain development in adolescence

A standout trait of the teenage years is the gradual shift toward independence, often called *social reorientation*, away from under the watchful eyes of parents and other adults. This natural progression is seen across the animal kingdom, where young mammals and fledgling birds eventually leave their dens and nests.

As adolescents grow, their social brain networks undergo significant structural and functional maturation, leading to patterns of neural activity that resemble those of adults. This development is closely linked to social reorientation.

As adolescents seek independence, the social world gains importance. Functional changes observed in teens' brains include:

>> Heightened sensitivity means they're more sensitive to social and emotional cues than adults.

>> Enhanced perception of social risks and a stronger desire for social rewards (which can sometimes be stronger than the desire for money).

>> With emerging cognitive skills, teenagers gradually get better at seeing situations from other people's points of view, which helps them understand others, control their emotions, and get along with their friends.

Social belonging and identity formation

The teenage years are a time of self-discovery and identity formation, when young people start to establish a sense of who they are, what they believe in, and where they fit into the world.

On the importance of belonging

Think back to your younger days when exclusion from a social event — a trip to a game, mall, or party — felt devastatingly painful. You might remember the sting of not being invited to the party or trip to the mall, being the subject of cruel gossip, or having notes passed around you weren't privy to. This behavior is especially prevalent among teenage girls who're more driven than boys to enforce a level social structure. Being left out strikes at the heart of the need to belong.

Developmental psychology research indicates that young people, especially in their early to mid-adolescence, heavily value the opinions of their peers. While younger children typically have a positive view of themselves, often described as high self-esteem, this perception changes during adolescence. Teens start to assess themselves more in terms of how they believe others see them. Furthermore, experiences of social rejection or exclusion tend to impact their mood more negatively than in adults over the age of 25.

Helping young people find their sense of self

Young people who don't develop a robust self-identity often face challenges with their confidence and may be more prone to taking risks and suffering from mental health problems such as anxiety and depression. On the other hand, teens with a well-established sense of self are in a better position to make sound decisions in life. They tend to choose healthier options and maintain a positive attitude. Additionally, they are more adept at dealing with difficulties, including peer pressure and the demands of school.

Here are some practical tips for parents on guiding teenagers toward a strong self-identity:

>> Encourage teens to identify and focus on their interests and goals to foster a clear sense of self.

>> Support teenagers in reflecting on their life and feelings through open, ongoing conversations.

>> Help teens learn to assertively say "no" when necessary to protect their time and self-respect.

>> Ensure teenagers feel accepted and affirmed to strengthen their self-esteem and ability to bounce back from challenges.

>> Teach teens positive self-talk and to recognize their own strengths and qualities.

>> Challenge and reject stereotypes and encourage teens to value and express their unique identities.

Assessing the Risk of Risky Business

Teens are usually stereotyped as reckless risk takers, self-centered, and highly sensitive to social pressure. And their "half-developed" or "offline" adolescent brains are usually blamed. That said, researchers are still looking for a framework to explain why risk-taking and sensation-seeking inclinations are more prevalent in adolescents than in children or adults.

Venting about the ventral striatum

The *ventral striatum*, including the NAcc, is a brain region associated with learning and processing risk versus reward. During the teenage years, brain imaging shows it's more sensitive and hyperreactive than in childhood or adulthood.

REMEMBER

One idea is that heightened ventral striatum sensitivity evolved to encourage adaptive behaviors such as exploration and curiosity — essential for having courage to leave the safety of the nest! The downside of these behaviors is the bravado that often leads young people toward daring (and sometimes dangerous) acts.

Risk-taking and peer approval

One way researchers have explored the interactions of risk-taking and social approval in the lab is with computer gaming. A classic 2005 study published in *Developmental Psychology* found that young teens, ages 13 to 16, engaged in riskier behaviors in a driving simulation when their friends were present. However, when they were driving alone, their risk-taking was as sensible as for adults. This finding suggests that teens have the cognitive capacity for sound judgment-making, but they're susceptible to *hot cognition*. This term describes decision-making processes that are heavily swayed by emotional states, such as the thrill of having an audience or the urge to impress others, highlighting how the presence of peers can significantly influence adolescents' propensity for risk.

Three theories of risk-taking

To understand why teenagers may take more risks when their friends are around, scientists have come up with a few different theories. Most likely all three are at play:

>> **Social Motivation Model:** This idea says that teens are motivated by the need to fit in with their friends (no kidding!). They make decisions based on what they think will help their peer group accept them. Tribe approval overrules sensibility at times.

>> **Reward Sensitivity Model:** This theory suggests that teens' brains are far more sensitive to rewards than adults' brains are. Because their self-regulation is still developing, they may take more risks if they think something fun or rewarding will happen.

>> **Value-Based Model:** This approach believes that teens weigh the importance of different choices based on what they value in the moment. If fitting in with friends is what they value most, they're more likely to take risks if they think it will make them seem cooler to their friends.

REMEMBER

Adolescent brain researchers now understand risky behavior is driven more by pleasure than by pain. Poor decision-making and risk-evaluation don't happen in isolation. The reward is clear: tribe approval.

Understanding the Ups and Downs of Mental Health Challenges in Teenagers

Feeling worried, sad, tearful, or stressed, is commonplace when you're going through puberty and your teenage years. Sometimes it's difficult to discern normal moodiness from a serious mental health problem. Learning how to regulate your emotional well-being is a key skill (hopefully) practiced and refined during adolescence.

WARNING

When sadness or worry is excessive or prolonged and interferes with everyday life such as school or socializing, this is a clear sign it's time to seek professional advice.

Common mental health problems in teens

Globally, adolescence is a vulnerable time for mental health problems. The WHO notes the most common mental health problems in adolescents include:

>> **Mood disorders:** Anxiety disorders are the most common, with a higher prevalence in older adolescents. Depression also becomes more frequent, and both can hinder school performance and increase isolation.

>> **Behavioral disorders:** ADHD and conduct disorders are found more often in younger adolescents (starting in early childhood).

>> **Eating disorders:** Disorders such as anorexia and bulimia often start during adolescence, with serious consequences including high mortality rates.

>> **Psychosis:** Symptoms such as hallucinations or delusions typically appear in late adolescence and can disrupt daily life and education. Psychosis is a strong risk factor for developing schizophrenia.

>> **Suicide and self-harm:** Suicide is a leading cause of death among adolescents, influenced by various factors including substance abuse and barriers to care.

Why are teens vulnerable to mental health problems?

To determine the age of onset of mental health disorders, a 2022 large-scale meta-analysis published in *Molecular Psychiatry* considered 192 studies involving 708,561 individuals. The study included neurodevelopmental disorders, mood disorders such as depression, anxiety, eating disorders, obsessive compulsive disorders, schizophrenia-spectrum disorders/primary psychotic, substance use disorders/addictive behavior, and personality disorders/related traits.

Here are the key findings:

>> Neurodevelopmental disorder onset (meaning ADHD and autism, which are usually first noticed in early childhood) typically peaks around the age of five and half.

>> Globally, about one-third of people experience their first mental health diagnosis by the age of 14, nearly half by the age of 18, and over half by the age of 25.

>> The peak age for the onset of all mental disorders is 14.5 years.

WARNING

The main take-away from this work is that mental health disorders emerge during adolescence. As I point out earlier in the chapter, a lot is changing during these years. But it's especially important to recognize this is when the brain is most plastic, perhaps pointing toward a vulnerability. Broadly speaking, the brain and nervous system are at their most vulnerable to stress and the emergence of problems during critical or sensitive periods.

However, as the authors of the 2022 study state, although mental health promotion, prevention, and early intervention can be implemented over the lifespan, ". . . the benefits are maximal when young people are targeted at around the time of onset of mental disorders."

Why poor mental health is sharply increasing

Since the mid 2010s, there's been a noticeable rise in depression, anxiety, and suicidality among adolescents worldwide. This trend accelerated during the COVID-19 pandemic. Various theories have been put forward to explain this dramatic increase.

COVID-19 pandemic and uncertainty

The COVID-19 pandemic magnified factors contributing to poor mental health, particularly social isolation and economic challenges. Adolescents especially struggled with the overwhelming uncertainty surrounding health, education, and social connections. The relationship between tolerance of uncertainty and teenage mental health shows that teens are more likely to have mental health problems if they didn't have the psychological tools or support to cope with "fear of the unknown."

Digital technology

Even before the pandemic, adolescent mental health was declining, raising questions about the role of digital technology. While screen time is often blamed, research shows mixed results. A 2024 Oxford study found that internet use could boost well-being, but the dark side of the internet — such as cyberbullying, online harassment, and social media pressures — can be harmful, particularly for girls. The connection between mental health and social media is complex, with research indicating it varies by individual and developmental stage.

REMEMBER

The problem is that as I'm writing this book, studies can't definitively say if social media use causes mental health issues or vice versa. And most researchers aren't yet willing to make policy recommendations and suggest interventions with certainty.

Prevention and early intervention work best

TIP

Preventing mental health issues and catching them early are the most effective strategies. It's so important to teach young people how to understand and manage their emotions, offer healthy alternatives to risky behaviors, and build strong, supporting communities with plenty of positive role models. Digital media, health services, schools, and community programs should all be tapped into especially to connect with help for the most at-risk teens.

As the WHO points out, instead of hospital stays and heavy psychiatric medication, the focus should shift to prevention. Prevention is better than the ambulance at the bottom of the cliff. By providing young people the tools and support, we can build a strong fence at the top of the cliff, ensuring they never fall in the first place!

Emphasizing Positive Brain Behaviors for Adolescent Brain Health

Teenagers' brains are amazing at changing and adapting — at their peak of plasticity, offering a unique chance to make a difference. Elsewhere in this book (Chapters 12 to 20), I explore the importance of nutrition, exercise, sleep, and other lifestyle choices in brain health. Here, I address a few key concerns about this phase of life that needs extra understanding and care.

The impact of substance use on developing brains

Teenagerhood is a paradox! Right around the exact time when teens are often most drawn to sensation-seeking and experimentation with mind-altering substances is when such substances can do the most harm to their developing brains. Alcohol, cannabis, and other mind-altering drugs pose significant risks and challenges.

WARNING

It's safest to keep all mind-altering substances and teenagers apart (but as a parent of teenagers, I'm aware this is easier said than done!).

Alcohol

The dangers of excess alcohol consumption in teenagers, are two-fold. Firstly, young people who drink are more likely to engage in dangerous behaviors that lead to serious injuries, for example, drunk driving, falls, or stumbling into oncoming traffic. Secondly, alcohol's neurotoxic effects can disrupt healthy development and exacerbate mental health problems.

Cannabis

According to the Centers for Disease Control (CDC) four in ten U.S. high school students reported having used cannabis at least once. The dangers for regular users are multifold. Firstly, regular users have difficulties with clear thinking, memory, learning, coordination, attention, and subsequent challenges with schoolwork. Secondly, users are less likely to graduate high school and attend college. Finally, use heightens the risk of mental health problems, including depression, social anxiety, and psychosis.

WARNING

The link between cannabis and long-lasting mental disorders such as schizophrenia is particularly strong in those who start using it early and frequently, a risk that's amplified for individuals with certain genetic profiles.

Cannabis use is illegal or limited to strictly medical purposes in many parts of the world. Despite the ongoing debate (often fueled by advocates of the substance) around cannabis's causal role in triggering psychosis and schizophrenia, the precautionary principle suggests a conservative approach for the adolescent brain.

WARNING

The advice is clear: If someone chooses to use cannabis, it is far safer to wait until both the person and their brain have reached adulthood.

Technology and the teenage brain

As technology evolves at a breakneck pace, young people possess the digital agility adults frequently lack. While kids effortlessly connect, learn, and game their way online, adults and experts worry about screen time and debate whether bans on phones in schools improve mental health and academic attainment. As mentioned earlier in the chapter, studies about cause and effect remain inconclusive.

Concerns about technology and the teenage brain usually center on three main areas, each with its own challenges and opportunities:

» **Devices:** Studies are exploring the way teenagers spend time on their devices, from the type of content consumed (such as, porn, mental health intervention apps, social media) to the duration (such as, how many hours per day), the timing of use (for example, during school or late at night), and the age and developmental stage of the device user. Rather than banning devices, digital health researchers advocate for digital literacy approaches.

» **Gaming:** Gaming holds a dual-edged sword; it has been linked to improved spatial navigation, reasoning, and problem-solving, and, for adolescent boys especially, is often a means of social connection. However, reasonable questions remain to be answered about the risks of bullying in online multiplayer gaming, gaming addiction, the role of violent games in promoting aggression, and whether screen time is displacing in-person interactions.

» **Social media:** Provides a platform for social connection and learning (and this is especially the case for young people who identify as minorities or with disability). But excessive use (especially in some younger adolescent girls and high school graduates) is associated with greater risks of anxiety, depression, and other mental health issues.

TIP

While research on the effects of device use, gaming and social media on adolescent mental health yields inconsistent findings, the consensus points to a slight negative correlation. But what makes one teenager resilient versus another vulnerable to the negative impacts of technology needs to be better understood before any clear advice can be given.

Teenage sleep schedules

Healthy sleep contributes to physical health, immune function, mental health, and academic performance. In Chapter 14, I go into detail about sleep. Sleep disturbance in adolescence is common and is driven by several factors including changes in sleep/wake timings (*chronotype*):

>> **Pubertal hormones:** Teenagers often experience a shift toward a more evening-oriented chronotype due to pubertal changes in *melatonin* (the sleep hormone) release. This shift corresponds to later sleep times (typically much later than their middle-aged parents!). In short, teenagers don't start to feel sleepier until much later in the evening.

>> **Devices:** While they're waiting to feel sleep, you can nearly guarantee they are exposing themselves to blue light from screens (such as, smartphones, computers, and TVs). Blue light exposure after the sun has gone down interferes with melatonin production, delaying sleep onset and reducing overall sleep duration.

>> **Early school start times:** Now the late-to-bed teenager needs to wake up early for school. The school bell conflicts with the natural shift toward later sleep times in teenagers, resulting in insufficient sleep during school days.

>> **Busy after-school schedules:** Homework, extracurricular activities, and social engagements (all of which parents and teachers encourage) can also lead to later bedtimes, further restricting sleep duration and affecting sleep quality.

>> **Social jetlag:** This factor describes the mismatch between the biological need for sleep and social obligations! It's compounded by the variations in sleep timing between work/school days and weekends or holidays. Social jetlag is particularly problematic in teenagers who like to stay up late on the weekend and then need to wake early for school on Monday.

Encouraging healthy risk-taking

Examples of positive risk-taking include engaging in competitive sports or outdoor adventure activities, which teach discipline, teamwork, and the handling of both success and failure. Daring to speak up in class or stepping into the spotlight on stage can work wonders for a young person's confidence. Similarly, channeling their energy into creative arts opens avenues for self-expression. And for those who take the lead on projects or clubs, even the small wins can foster a quiet, yet profound, sense of pride.

It all sounds a little clichéd, and as a parent of teenagers, I know how often adults are told they are "cringe" or ignored or eye-rolled! Encouraging young people to take calculated chances is crucial for their growth and self-discovery, not panicking about what may go wrong. Good luck!

Supporting adolescents through storm and stress

For parents, caregivers, and other adults who work with young people, creating a space for conversations and the exchange of thoughts and personal stories is crucial. This relationship-building is especially significant into the teenage years, a time when they particularly need parental advice and support but often don't want to ask.

AN EXAMPLE OF GOOD TIMING: ADOLESCENCE AND HIGH SCHOOL EDUCATION

In an interesting twist, U.K. researchers once asked 85 teenagers for their take on the neuroscientific view of their developmental stage. Remarkably, many were uninterested, calling it boring or even intrusive, believing it dehumanized them and eroded their autonomy (though not to me as a neuroscientist and mother of teenagers). While other teenagers acknowledged that knowing the teenage perspective could help to dispel myths and fight stereotypes, one questioned the difference in curiosity researchers have between adolescent and adult brains.

The young people who participated in the survey were smart enough to see the potential for neuroscience research but felt it could be better used to obtain insights and understanding into teen behavior without the usual load of moral judgment and stereotyping.

REMEMBER

Some adults seem to find both humor and horror in the concept of the adolescent brain. Somehow, you may forget about the positive outcomes that can result from owning and operating such adaptable neural circuitry. In my experience, young people are wonderfully compassionate, empathic, and devoted friends, they're often highly motivated and goal-oriented, and they're at their peak of their learning potential and creativity.

The young people I know stand on the cusp of greatness; and with a nudge in the right direction, a bit of patience, and the right opportunities, you can watch them soar to heights. So, let's invest a little more faith and a lot more support in our teenagers, for they are not just primed for success — they're already on their way there.

IN THIS CHAPTER

» Exploring longevity trends and their causes

» Reframing midlife's challenges and opportunities

» Aging's impact on brain structure and function

» Key biological markers of aging

» Distinguishing normal memory changes from dementia signs

Chapter **8**

Supporting Healthy Brain Aging

Aging is inevitable and happens to everyone.

There is little doubt that, in much of the world, we now live decades longer than our ancestors ever did. But the question is, if humans are living longer, how do aging brains fare? Dementia, memory loss, and cognitive decline are strongly associated with aging, and Alzheimer's disease is one of the major causes of death worldwide. So, is the payoff for living a longer life memory loss and poor brain function in the latter years?

In this chapter, you consider the various aspects of aging and how it relates to brain health. You examine trends in longevity and investigate their underlying causes, reframing midlife's challenges as opportunities for growth and adaptation. Additionally, you discover how aging impacts brain structure and function, discuss key biological markers of aging, and differentiate between normal memory changes and signs of dementia.

Living to 100: Modern Trends in Aging

More and more people are living into very old age, and there has never been a better time in which to do so. Thanks to humanity's intelligence, modern medicine and socioeconomic mobility has enabled us to manage reproductive health, avoid maternal and neonatal death, vaccinate against disease, prevent pain, treat infection and some cancers, and perform surgery if required. One hundred years ago, few people lived barely long enough to see out their 50s. A baby born today in a wealthy country can expect to live to see out the first decades of the 22nd century.

Defining aging

How do you define aging? Is it when you start feeling "old"? And if so, are you old?

There are many academic definitions and perspectives of aging. In sum, most state aging is not just as a biological decline, but a biological, psychological, social, and cultural phenomenon. Biologically, aging affects your cells and tissues, everything from slowing metabolism to your cells' ability to regenerate and repair. This natural and irreversible process varies widely — some people age gracefully, others find it challenging, and for some, it involves health complications. Psychologically, aging challenges your perceived capabilities and limits — attitudes toward getting older (self and others) can range from acceptance to resistance. Culturally, aging affects how the world sees you and the roles you play within your family and community.

Aging as a disease

Thanks to longevity science, it's become popular in recent times to state, "Aging is a disease." In 2022, there was debate whether or not to add "old age" into the 11th revision of the WHO International Classification of Diseases, thus defining it as a condition that could be treated or cured.

Defining longevity

Discussions of aging and longevity include a few terms that sound interchangeable, but have specific meanings:

» **Life expectancy:** The average number of years a person is expected to live based on statistical factors like birth year and location.

» **Lifespan:** The maximum length of time an individual of a species can live, with humans reaching up to 122 years.

>> **Healthspan:** The period during which a person remains healthy and free from serious illness, usually shorter than lifespan.

>> **Longevity:** Living significantly beyond the average life expectancy, often under ideal conditions.

Queen Elizabeth II is an excellent example of someone whose *healthspan* closely matched their *lifespan*. The Queen maintained a robust state of health, and was reportedly "bright and focused," fulfilling her royal duties including meeting the new British prime minister a mere two days before she died in 2022.

Perceiving age and ageism

Ageism refers to stereotypes, prejudice, and discrimination based on age. It can impact how you feel about yourself and how others treat you. For example, older people may avoid bright colors to not appear "trying too hard," or younger workers may dismiss older colleagues' ideas.

The 2021 Global Report on Ageism found that half the world holds ageist views, which harms older adults' health, leads to cognitive decline, and worsens isolation.

Aging populations: People worldwide are living longer

In 1800, a newborn baby could expect to live for around 32 years (and no region in the world had a life expectancy over 40). But by 2021, a baby born anywhere on the planet could expect to live to 71 years. In many regions of the world, the life expectancy of a newborn today is over 80.

REMEMBER

Life expectancy has increased steadily over the past 50 years. So much so, global life expectancy increased about four to five months per calendar year!

But where, when, how, and why did this big change happen? According to The World in Data, it's a common misconception that life expectancy has only increased because of declines in child mortality. But this isn't the full story. High child mortality contributed significantly to short lifespans in the past, and it has declined, but people of all ages can expect to live longer. Fewer babies, children, middle-aged adults, and older people are dying than in the past. For example, I'm nearly 50 and live in Australia. In 1900, I could expect to live to about 70, but today I could expect to live to 83. A gain of 13 years.

LIFE EXPECTANCY IN THE UNITED STATES

The United States is a life-expectancy outlier. Americans have a lower life expectancy than people in other rich countries. Life expectancy in the U.S. is around 78. In comparison, countries such as Australia, Japan, Spain, and Sweden all have life expectancies of over 83. According to the World in Data, Americans suffer higher death rates from smoking, obesity, homicides, opioid overdoses, suicides, road accidents, and infant deaths. In addition to this, deeper poverty and less access to healthcare mean Americans die at a younger age than poor people in other rich countries.

REMEMBER

This huge shift in life expectancy has come about from advances in the following: nutrition, clean water, sanitation, neonatal healthcare, antibiotics, vaccines, and other technologies and public health efforts — and improvements in living standards, economic growth, and poverty reduction. Even today, differences in life expectancy between countries are due to differences in wealth and healthcare; for example, in 2021, Nigeria's life expectancy was 30 years lower than Japan's.

TECHNICAL STUFF

Thanks to the COVID-19 pandemic, life expectancy in many countries dipped for the first time since World War II (as of 2024, it's now bouncing back). Deaths among those over 60 drove this. Australia, New Zealand, Norway, and Denmark were the few countries that continued to show increases in life expectancy in the first two years of the pandemic.

Connecting with Centenarians

Once rare as diamonds, the oldest of the old are the fastest growing sector of the global population. If you were born in 1900, your chances of living to be 100 were fewer than one in a million, and few people lived until the 1950s. For females born in wealthy nations today, the chances of blowing out 100 candles on a cake are about one in fifty!

Studying centenarians

Because of the deep curiosity about their secrets to longevity, centenarians have been the focus of plenty of research. The Japanese Okinawa Centenarian Study, started by Dr. Makoto Suzuki back in 1975 is the longest-running study.

THE OLDEST PERSON EVER

On February 21, 1875, one year before Bell filed his patent for the telephone, a baby girl, Jeanne Louise Calment was born in Arles, France. She was alive to witness the invention of the airplane, cinema, and on a trip to Paris saw the Eiffel tower being built. When she was 13, Jeanne met Vincent Van Gogh, although apparently, she was less than impressed, saying he was "...very ugly, ungracious, impolite..."

In 1997, the same year Princess Diana died, Calment finally passed away. She was 122 years and 164 days old. Although blind, almost deaf, and confined to a wheelchair, Calment reportedly remained spirited and "alert as a hummingbird" till the end. The French called her *"la doyenne de l'humanité"* (the elder of humankind) and she still holds the record for the world's longest-ever living human.

Once recruited, centenarians — or any other older person participating in an aging study — have their age verified (sometimes it turns out they're not as old as claimed!) and they are assessed for mental, physical, cognitive, and social health. Some undergo blood tests, brain scans, or even join brain donation programs. To add individual anecdotes and richness to the study an autobiographical interview is usually conducted. Given the relative scarcity of extremely old folks, many groups from around the globe have pooled their resources and data to enable more powerful conclusions to be drawn.

Zoning in on the Blue Zones

Another longevity research made well-known by *National Geographic* writer Dan Buettner is The Blue Zones. Although there's controversy around the validity of the actual ages of some "Blue Zones" residents, they typically remain in good health as they age, and we can take plenty from their lifestyle choices.

Blue Zones residents share nine specific characteristics:

>> **Move naturally:** No gyms or marathons here. Blue Zones residents move through daily activities like gardening and housework.

>> **Purpose:** The Okinawans call it "Ikigai" and the Nicoyans call it "plan de vida." Having a clear "why" to wake up adds up to seven years of life expectancy.

>> **Downshift:** They reduce stress with daily rituals, like prayer, naps, or happy hour.

>> **80 percent rule:** "Hara hachi bu" or stop eating when 80-percent full and eat smaller meals later in the day.

>> **Plant slant:** Diets are rich in beans with meat served sparingly, about five times a month.

>> **Wine at 5:** People in all blue zones (except Adventists) drink alcohol moderately and regularly. Moderate drinkers outlive non-drinkers.

>> **Belong:** Being part of a faith-based community adds years to life expectancy.

>> **Loved ones first:** Family is a priority. They keep parents nearby, commit to partners, and invest in children.

>> **Right tribe:** They surround themselves with friends who reinforce healthy habits.

TECHNICAL STUFF

The idea of blue zones originated from a demographic study by Gianni Pes and Michel Poulain published in the *Journal of Experimental Gerontology*, which showed Sardinia, Italy, to have a large concentration of very old, very healthy people. Using a blue Bic marker pen, Pes and Poulain drew concentric rings around these incredibly long-living Sardinian communities. As such, Pes, Poulain, and Buettner started calling these communities the "Blue Zones."

Surviving, escaping, or delaying diseases of aging

Longevity researchers with the New England Centenarian Study (NECS) have identified three broad groups of centenarians: Escapers, Delayers, and Survivors, so named because of their routes to avoid the major age-related diseases that kill off their peers. The diseases of aging they typically avoid include cancer, stroke, heart attack, diabetes, and dementia.

>> **Escapers** are those very lucky people who have managed to escape illness altogether and are living till 100 with remarkably strong mental and physical capabilities.

>> **Delayers** tend to delay any age-related illness until their late 80s.

>> **Survivors** are those people who have been diagnosed with an age-related disease before 80 and yet survive.

NECS found that for every five centenarians, one was an Escaper, two were Survivors and two were Delayers. Even though men were far less likely to reach 100, they were twice as likely to be Escapers than women. Men and women were equally likely to be Survivors or Delayers.

Learning lessons from centenarians

One consistent theme emerging from the longevity research is that genetics contributes about 30 percent to longevity, while lifestyle factors account for the remaining 70 percent. Depending on the study you read, these percentages vary somewhat (sometimes 80:20, other times 75:25, but that ratio is the general range). A healthy lifestyle includes maintaining a balanced diet, regular exercise, and staying socially active. Among the most significant findings is the importance of personality traits such as resilience, adaptability, and optimism. Many centenarians cite optimism as a lifelong characteristic significantly influencing their longevity.

Some centenarians retain cognitive prowess

Some centenarians often remain cognitively intact and "sharp as a tack," suggesting that cognitive decline isn't inevitable at extreme old ages.

One study of 340 Dutch centenarians found their cognitive performance remained stable through their 80s, 90s, and 100s. Despite the presence of AD-associated neuropathology and exposure to risk factors such as smoking, healthy centenarians maintain their cognitive functioning even after their 100th birthday, with only a slight decline in memory function, suggesting some resilience or resistance against factors that usually contribute to decline.

This resilience is sometimes attributed to cognitive reserve (which I explain more in Chapter 16). In short, people possess a sort of neural resilience through good genes or a lifetime of rich cognitive training, allowing for higher levels of brain degeneration before any clinical symptoms appear. Factors such as education, cognitive activity frequency, and higher IQ are associated with cognitive reserve in centenarians.

Does longevity run in families?

Everyone probably has the genetic capability to live to at least their 80s. This makes sense in the context of results from the study of Seventh Day Adventists at Loma Linda University who live eight to ten years longer than the average American. They tend to be physically fit, vegetarian, and non-smokers, who spend a lot of time with their families and their church group. The New England Centenarian Study (NECS) team, who studied the church-going group, state the average American has the genes to reach their mid-late 80s; they just need to take very good care of themselves with proper lifestyle choices.

Exceptional longevity runs in families — the children and siblings of centenarians are healthier, have a more favorable "biological signature," and they age slower than their peers. Tellingly, Jeanne Calment's brother Francois lived till the age of 97, but as she put it, "God didn't want there to be two 100-year-olds in the same family, so it fell to me."

TIP

That said, most experts agree that good genes will only get you so far.

Minding yourself in midlife

The Dunedin Multidisciplinary Health and Development Study has meticulously tracked just over 1,000 people born in the 1970s in Dunedin, New Zealand, who are now in their early 50s. The team started to see differences in aging trajectories of aging emerge in the group by the time they were in their 30s. They identified three aging patterns:

>> An average group who experienced one year of physiological decline per calendar year.

>> A fastest-aging group who experienced more than twice this rate of change.

>> A slow-aging group who experienced almost no change at all per calendar year.

Biological aging was estimated by charting the decline of cardiovascular, metabolic, endocrine, lung, liver, kidney, renal, immune, and dental health biomarkers. Factors such as family longevity, social class, childhood adversity, health, intelligence, and self-control were linked to accelerated aging in the fast-aging group.

WARNING

Because these differences in the rate of aging emerged when the study members were in their early 30s, it's essential to start examining how you might prevent aging earlier in life. Think of midlife as more opportunity than crisis!

Charting Healthy Trajectories of Brain Aging

It should come as no surprise that as your hair greys, you develop wrinkles, your joints start to ache, and your brain also changes with age. The brain's structure, function and mental capabilities change, and usually (but not always) start a slow steady decline from around age 30. But the rate of change varies person to person.

Cellular hallmarks of aging

Because aging is a complex process, chronological age doesn't accurately show how biological processes change or how people differ. This is the reason that scientists are now examining biological indicators or hallmarks of cellular aging and monitoring their changes over time.

When the hallmarks of aging were first published in 2013, they included. DNA instability, telomere attrition, epigenetic alterations, loss of proteostasis, deregulated nutrient-sensing, mitochondrial dysfunction, cellular senescence, stem cell exhaustion, and altered intercellular communication. The list has now expanded to include disabled macro autophagy, chronic inflammation, and dysbiosis. The great hope of aging science is to medically target each hallmark to improve healthspan and lifespan.

WARNING

Telomeres rightly generate excitement as markers of aging because they shorten each time a cell divides, potentially leading to cell aging or death. However, this doesn't apply to neurons in the brain, which are post-mitotic meaning they do not divide after they are born. So, neurons maintain their telomere length over time, as there is no division to cause them to shorten, making telomeres a less critical factor in the aging of neurons!

Understanding the markers of brain aging

Brain aging is marked by changes in grey matter volume, white matter integrity, and network connectivity, which professionals use to assess aging relative to your chronological age.

While some mild cognitive slowing and brain atrophy are normal in healthy aging, unhealthy aging includes rapid decline, often leading to Alzheimer's disease. The trick is differentiating between the two! This is where the professionals you met in Chapter 3 come in. They're crucial for diagnosis and tailoring care and interventions.

Healthy aging affects brain structure

After age 35, brain volume loss becomes more pronounced, with an annual decline of around 0.2 percent to 0.5 percent. The rate of atrophy accelerates further after the age of 60, with a steady volume loss exceeding 0.5 percent per year. Different brain regions may experience varying degrees of atrophy (see Figure 8-1), with the frontal lobes typically showing the most significant shrinkage. Some of the typical markers noted in brain scans include:

>> **Brain atrophy:** Progressive frontal and parietal atrophy predict the level of brain aging. Atrophy shows up as grey matter and white matter volume loss, cortical thinning, sulci deepening and widening, and gyri loss.

>> **Ventricular enlargement:** As brain tissue shrinks, the ventricles, or fluid-filled spaces within the brain, become larger. This is an indirect sign of surrounding brain tissue shrinkage.

>> **White matter hyperintensities:** These spots of increased brightness in the brain's white matter associated with vascular (blood vessel) changes and ischemia (oxygen deprivation) in the aging brain. Their severity correlates with age and brain function decline.

>> **Cerebral microhemorrhages:** Increase with age and are linked to cognitive decline.

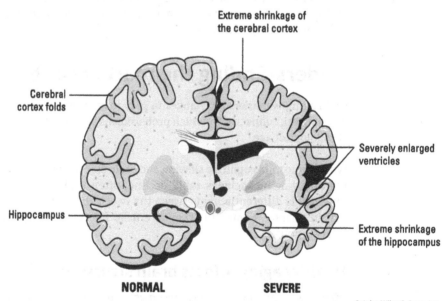

Extreme shrinkage of the cerebral cortex

Cerebral cortex folds

Severely enlarged ventricles

Hippocampus

Extreme shrinkage of the hippocampus

NORMAL   SEVERE

© John Wiley & Sons, Inc.

FIGURE 8-1:
A healthy young brain (left) and an aging brain (right) with severe atrophy.

Healthy brain aging under the microscope

Degenerative diseases such as AD result from the death of neurons. But in a healthy aging brain, there is hardly any cell death. Instead, brain shrinkage comes from other factors affecting neurons and glia.

» In grey matter, the density of dendritic arbors and dendrites spines decreases, resulting in overall brain volume loss.

» Levels of enzymes that synthesize neurotransmitters decline with age. These changes, combined with decreased synaptic plasticity, reduced dendritic branching, and altered gene expression in neurons, make the brain less efficient overall.

» Neurons have limited capacity to regeneration, but there's evidence glia do renew themselves. But as you age, oligodendrocyte precursor cells (OPCs) and myelin renewal age, too.

» Neuroinflammation is associated with microglia and astrocytes. As you age, there is an increase in pro-inflammatory cytokines and chemokines, as well as an increase in reactive oxygen species (ROS) and oxidative stress, which can damage neurons and other cells.

» The blood-brain barrier (BBB) is a specialized barrier that separates the blood from the brain. It's composed of endothelial cells (ECs) and other cells, and it regulates the exchange of molecules between the blood and the brain. As you age, there are changes in the BBB, including decreased tight junction proteins, increased permeability, and increased inflammation. These changes can lead to the accumulation of toxic molecules in the brain and contribute to neuro-degenerative diseases.

Cognitive changes expected with aging

One interesting and encouraging finding is that while some cognitive functions decline with age others don't! Cognitive skills such as working memory, verbal fluency (for example, naming 25 objects starting with a certain letter) and visuo-spatial abilities (such as, arranging blocks into patterns or drawing a 3D object) tend to decline with age. But the good news is skills such as vocabulary and comprehension show minimal decline and may even improve in midlife! More on this idea later in the chapter.

Healthy aging affects cognitive networks

In healthy young people, specialized nodes in the brain are responsible for managing specific tasks with different nodes cost-effectively and rapidly communicating with others. Network function is another measure of brain aging. Three fMRI measures of healthy brain aging include:

» The HAROLD effect (Hemispheric Asymmetry Reduction in OLder aDults) measures age-related "balance" or asymmetry of connectivity between the left and right prefrontal cortex (PFC) during cognitive tests. Older adults show less lop-sidedness versus younger adults.

>> The PASA model (Posterior-Anterior Shift in Aging) measures age-related shifts in occipital lobe (posterior) activity versus in frontal lobe (anterior) activity. Older adults show more frontal and less occipital activity versus younger adults.

>> Network segregation/integration of aging measures processing in specialized brain nodes (that is, segregation) but also cooperation between different nodes (that is, integration). Older adults show less segregation and more integration.

REMEMBER

A healthy human brain operates on the "less is more" principle, prioritizing efficiency and energy conservation. When learning a new skill, your brain initially expends a lot of energy, but as you master the skill, it uses less and less. As you age, however, the brain's efficiency declines, and it compensates by activating more networks and connections, much like a team that starts to rely on every member to contribute to heavy tasks instead of just a few. This increased recruitment across the brain helps offset the effects of aging.

Healthy aging affects activities of daily life

Functional markers provide insights into how aging affects various brain processes such as thinking, feeling, and behaving:

>> **Cognitive function:** Cognitive abilities such as memory, language, and judgment typically decline with age. Specific changes in episodic memory and processing speed are significant indicators of brain aging.

>> **Motor coordination:** Aging affects fine motor skills or dexterity, such as writing with a pen or buttoning a shirt.

>> **Sensory perception:** Sensory abilities such as vision and hearing degrade with age but well before brain aging sets in. In contrast, loss of smell or changes in olfaction are associated with brain dysfunction.

>> **Emotion:** Increases in anxiety and changes in emotional control are noted with aging but are influenced by overall health and psychological factors.

TECHNICAL
STUFF

DETECTING BRAIN AGING

Components of plasma, urine, and cerebrospinal fluid (CSF) are indispensable biomarkers for the assessment of brain aging. Changes that may be detected with aging include:

- **Tau protein:** Increases in tau protein, particularly its phosphorylated form (p-tau), are linked to tau pathologies such as Alzheimer's disease. These proteins accumulate with age and are associated with neurofibrillary tangles.

- **Neurofilament Light Chain (NfL):** This structural protein of neurons is a marker of neural damage and can predict cognitive decline as its levels increase in body fluids with age.

- **Glial Fibrillary Acidic Protein (GFAP):** Found in astrocytes, GFAP levels rise with age and are involved in various brain processes including synaptic formation. Elevated levels can indicate brain aging.

Knowing What's Normal: Aging Versus Dementia

Understanding the various memory and mental skills and what to expect as you age is crucial to knowing when to worry and seek help versus what is healthy and normal for your age.

Differentiating different types of cognitive skills and memories

Some of your mental skills may get a bit rusty as you age, while others stay the same and some even improve. That's because the different types of mental skills show different aging trajectories.

Crystallized and fluid mental skills

One useful way scientists have grouped these skills is into crystallized and fluid abilities (sometimes called "intelligences"):

>> **Crystallized abilities** are the skills, knowledge, and expertise you accumulated over your lifetime. For example, knowing that Paris is the capital of France.

>> **Fluid abilities** involve the capacity to think logically and solve problems in novel situations independent of your expertise or knowledge. It's your ability to analyze situations, identify patterns, and make logical connections between new information. For example, fixing a home repair by using logical thinking and problem-solving skills (versus calling a repairman).

Fluid and crystallized intelligence depend on different brain networks. Fluid intelligence is linked to regions like the PFC, while crystallized intelligence is tied to memory areas such as the hippocampus.

Different mental abilities peak at different ages (or do they?)

Have you ever encountered those magazine articles listing the ages at which different skills or talents peak? This topic can be inspiring (or deflating if that age is behind you) but studying cognitive abilities across ages turns out to be quite tricky.

However, studying how cognitive abilities change over time is more complex than it seems. Researchers use different study methods — some assess different age groups at one time, while others follow individuals over the years. These studies reveal mixed findings: some show that there's no single peak age, while others suggest specific skills peak at different times — like working memory around age 18 and vocabulary around age 60. Studies following the same people tend to show more stable patterns, with fluid abilities peaking in your 20s and 30s, then gradually declining, while crystallized abilities — like vocabulary — continue to grow with age and life experience.

TIP

Think of it like this: An 80-year-old today may not navigate a digital device nearly as adeptly as an 18-year-old. Would that mean they're less cognitive able? Or would a more reasonable measure be a longitudinal study that compares the 80-year-old to their younger self.

More generally, fluid abilities peak in your 20s and 30s and gradually decline after that. Crystallized abilities continue to increase throughout life with more education, intellectual engagement, and life experience, showing minimal decline even in late adulthood.

TIP

I like to think of crystalized abilities as wisdom, reflecting the culmination of knowledge and understanding acquired over a lifetime. However, in today's fast-paced society, where fluid abilities and speed often take precedence over deliberation, the value of wisdom, considered thought, and accumulated expertise may be overlooked.

Individual variation in cognitive decline

REMEMBER

Keep in mind that most research studies are based on averages drawn from hundreds, sometimes thousands, of individuals. While averages are useful, they don't capture individual differences. Consider the people you know, or even famous individuals — everyone ages at a different pace. Famously, Sophocles is said to have written *Oedipus at Colonus* when he was 92. And Sir David Attenborough, the

British broadcaster and natural historian, filmed and narrated the wildlife documentary *Planet Earth III* at 97.

Each person's aging trajectory is unique. Imagine if you were to administer a series of cognitive tests annually to three different individuals starting at age 70. You would likely see varying rates of change among them, as shown in Figure 8-2.

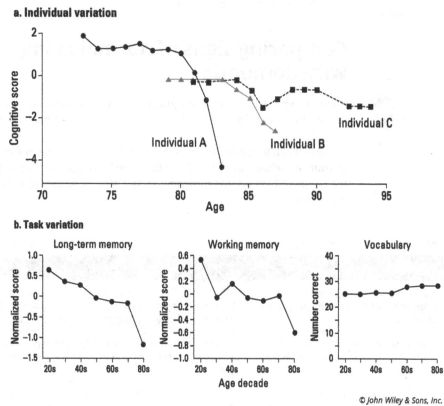

FIGURE 8-2: Variation in age-related cognitive decline.

© *John Wiley & Sons, Inc.*

These differences are influenced by many factors including a lucky dose of good genes and all the lifestyle factors outlined later in this book.

Making the most of midlife

Step away from the world of cognitive testing for a moment and consider what happens in the world of grown-up problem-solving and cognitive performance.

While your cognitive test scores might dip slightly in midlife, your real-world problem-solving skills often improve, thanks to life experience — what we can call wisdom! In many professions like surgery, law, or finance, practical experience becomes far more valuable than a high score on fluid intelligence. Wouldn't you prefer a seasoned expert for your heart surgery or financial advice over someone with just textbook knowledge?

REMEMBER

While younger people learn new skills quickly and effortlessly, midlife, and older adults excel in efficiency and competence in areas where they have honed their skills and expertise over the years.

Comparing signs of normal aging with dementia

TIP

Knowing what's normal for an aging brain can be reassuring, especially when differentiating these from signs that can suggest a condition such as dementia.

Because it can be confusing to know what to do if you spot one or more symptoms in yourself or someone else, The Alzheimer's Association has helpfully published ten signs and symptoms of dementia and also examples of normal aging, which you can see in Table 8-1.

TABLE 8-1   **Ten Examples of Normal Aging Versus Dementia**

Normal Aging	Worrying Signs of Dementia
Sometimes forgetting names or appointments but remembering them later	Disruptions in daily life due to memory loss, such as forgetting important dates or events, asking the same questions repeatedly, and increasingly needing to rely on memory aids
Making occasional mistakes when managing finances or household bills	Challenges in planning or solving problems — for example, struggling to remember monthly expenses or follow a well-known recipe
Occasionally needing help to use microwave settings or to record a TV show	Difficulty completing familiar tasks — for example, driving to a familiar location, organizing a grocery list, or remembering the rules of a favorite game
Getting confused about the day of the week but figuring it out later on	Losing track of dates, seasons, and the passage of time — for example, having trouble understanding something if it is not happening immediately or forgetting where they are or how they got there
Vision changes related to cataracts	Trouble understanding visual images and spatial relationships — for example, trouble reading, driving, or judging distance
Sometimes having trouble finding the right word	New problems with words in speaking or writing or having trouble with keeping up conversations — for example, repeating themselves or using the wrong names for people or things

Normal Aging	Worrying Signs of Dementia
Misplacing items from time to time, such as glasses or keys, but you can retrace your steps to find them	Misplacing items and losing the ability to retrace steps, often accusing others of stealing, especially as the disease progresses
Making a bad decision or mistake occasionally, such as neglecting to change the oil in the car	Changes in judgment or decision-making, using poor judgment when dealing with money or paying less attention to grooming or keeping themselves clean
Sometimes feeling uninterested in family or social obligations	Withdrawal from work or social activities
Becoming very "set in your ways" of doing things and becoming irritable when a routine is disrupted	Changes in mood and personality, becoming confused, suspicious, depressed, fearful, or anxious

REMEMBER

Memory loss is not always a sign of dementia! An example of normal forgetfulness is misplacing your car keys. A person with dementia, however, may lose their car keys and when they find them, forget what keys are used for.

REMEMBER

Feeling unsure or anxious about talking to others about these changes is normal. It may feel more "real" to express concerns about your own health. Or you can be afraid to anger someone by bringing up observations regarding changes in their skills or demeanor. If it's nothing serious, you can set your mind at ease; if it's something other than dementia, you may be able to start receiving treatment; and if it's a dementia diagnosis, the sooner you know, the more you can do.

Mild cognitive impairment (MCI)

There is, if I may use such a term, a grey area between normal aging-related cognitive changes and more obvious problems that could be dementia. Symptoms of mild cognitive impairment (MCI) are more noticeable than those linked to normal aging, but less severe than dementia symptoms.

TIP

While MCI indicates that your thinking and memory are impacted, your daily activities are not enough impacted to qualify as dementia. Someone with MCI breeze through daily tasks such as making a cup of tea or chatting on the phone, while maybe struggling a bit more with their finances or solving the Sunday crossword. While termed "mild" relative to dementia, MCI can still significantly impact a person and their family, making it a concerning health issue.

Diagnosing MCI

Because MCI can result from various factors, its important to rule these symptoms out. Diagnosing MCI involves a thorough review of medical history and cognitive testing, often requiring the exclusion of other conditions. In some parts of the world MCI is diagnosed by a specialist working in a memory clinic. Elsewhere your family doctor may be equipped to make a diagnosis.

Testing for MCI

One common tool that your family doctors may use to "grade" people on their current cognitive status and mental ability is the Mini Mental State Exam (MMSE). MMSE tests various cognitive domains including orientation to time and place, immediate and short-term recall, attention and calculation, language abilities, and visual-spatial skills. You may be asked for the date or the address you're living in. A doctor may hold up a pencil and their watch and ask you to name them. You may be asked to spell "WORLD" backwards or remember three items. Your MMSE scores a maximum of 30 points.

>> A score of 24 to 30 points is generally considered normal.

>> Scores below 24 may indicate some level of cognitive impairment and typically warrant further investigation.

>> Scores between 18 and 23 often indicate mild cognitive impairment.

>> Scores below 18 points suggest moderate to severe cognitive impairment.

Other tests or commonly used screening tools in clinical practice include the Montreal Cognitive Assessment (MoCA Test) and the General Practitioner Assessment of Cognition (GPCOG). Some countries have developed tools relevant to their population needs. For example, in Australia, the Kimberley Indigenous Cognitive Assessment (KICA-Cog) is the first cognitive assessment tool developed for use in remote Indigenous Australian populations.

WARNING

It's important to realize that these tests are screening tools and have limitations. If you're experiencing subtle cognitive changes, which are often called "brain fog" or simply "forgetfulness," these may not score below the typical threshold of concern (for example, below 24 points on MMSE) for dementia or MCI. This doesn't mean your "brain fog" isn't real, rather it's not necessarily indicative of a serious problem.

Treating MCI

Currently, there is no medical treatment (like a pill or surgery) for MCI. People should try lifestyle interventions such as regular exercise, a nutritious diet, mental stimulation, social engagement, and proper management of other health issues (for example, heart disease or diabetes). Regular monitoring and reassessment of cognitive functions are crucial for managing this condition.

While not all cases of MCI progress to dementia, individuals with MCI are at a higher risk of developing dementia and AD compared to their peers. But predicting who'll progress to the next state is particularly tricky. One study found around 13 percent of people with MCI progressed to dementia within three years. The good news here is most people didn't, so progression is not inevitable.

Monitoring your own memory

WARNING

It's not recommended you self-administer tools such as the MMSE. Firstly, memory loss and dementia can be mimicked by other health conditions, so sound clinical judgment is needed. Secondly, cognitive testing may be upsetting and it's better to avoid the burden of dealing with a distressed loved one by involving a doctor than going it alone. Finally, cognitive tests are subject to training effects. Training effects mean the more times you sit the test, the better you score. If you give your family members the test at home a few times, they may not show impairment when tested later on by their doctor. This preliminary test may delay diagnosis and access to support services.

WARNING

Despite your temptation, I urge you to have a doctor or other health care expert administer the MMSE or GPCOG.

In the meantime, here are a couple of online tools designed for you to monitor your own memory or that of a loved one. They both provide a report you can take to your doctor.

>> **BrainTrack** is a tool developed by Dementia Australia to help you track changes in your cognition every month using rather entertaining, travel-themed games. BrainTrack is available online at www.dementia.org.au/braintrack.

>> **Self-Administered Gerocognitive Exam (SAGE)** is designed to detect early signs of thinking, memory and cognition. You can SAGE yourself, or have family or friends take the test. SAGE is available online at https://braintest.com.

Demystifying Dementia and Alzheimer's Disease (AD)

Dementia is not a normal part of aging. Dementia is an umbrella term used to describe the symptoms of different diseases that cause a progressive decline in a person's memory and cognitive abilities.

Defining dementia

Symptoms of dementia vary from person to person. According to Dementia Australia, dementia can affect your:

>> **Memory:** You may find it harder to remember recent events, names of things, and people. It may also get harder to make new memories.

>> **Thinking:** You may get more confused, have trouble concentrating, planning, and problem-solving, struggle to complete everyday tasks, find it hard to think of the right word or express yourself, and find it hard to judge distances, directions, and time.

>> **Mood:** You may find yourself feeling less motivated and social, more prone to depression, anxiety, and agitation, or otherwise not yourself.

>> **Behavior:** You may start saying or doing things that are out of character for you. You may become restless and wander and have more disturbed sleep.

Over 100 diseases cause dementia symptoms including AD, Frontotemporal Dementia (FTD), vascular dementia, Parkinson's disease, Dementia with Lewy bodies, Huntington's disease, alcohol-related dementia (Korsakoff's syndrome), chronic traumatic encephalopathy (CTE), and Creutzfeldt-Jacob disease. Also, a variety of health issues, including depression, infections, brain tumors, vitamin deficiencies, and even menopause show some of these symptoms, which is why (I'll say it again!), a healthcare professional is invaluable for diagnosis and treatment.

Because AD is the most common form of dementia and accounts for 60-80 percent of dementia cases, the two terms are often used interchangeably (even though it isn't entirely accurate to do so).

REMEMBER

AD is a specific brain disease. AD is marked by symptoms of dementia that gradually get worse over time. Check out Chapter 4 for a brief overview of AD. The rest of this chapter provides information on the risks and possible prevention of AD.

Reducing your risk: There's good news

There is a good news story when it comes to AD risk! In many parts of the world your absolute risk of developing AD is lower now than it was 30 years ago. Recall in Chapter 5 I talked about why it's (absolutely) essential to consider your absolute risk. Here is why:

A comprehensive study published in 2020, which tracked the health of nearly 50,000 individuals over the age of 65, revealed that the rate of new dementia cases diagnosed in Europe and North America *decreased* by 13 percent per decade over the last 25 years. The total number of people living with the disease is increasing, but this is primarily due to more people living into old age — and age is the most significant risk factor.

The researchers suggest a few likely reasons for the decrease. Firstly, decades of improved heart disease management may have had a knock-on effect on brain health. We know a healthy heart correlates with a healthy brain (more on this later in the book in Chapter 13). However, it remains to be seen exactly which treatment — targeting inflammation, cholesterol, or blood pressure — has had the most significant impact on AD. Secondly, there is the availability and quality of formal education. Again, there is a correlation between years of education and AD risk (and more on that in Chapter 16). Consider that the average person born in the early 1900s left school once they hit their teens, people growing up in the latter half of last century stayed at school or headed off to college.

Taking action on your modifiable risk factors

Think of modifiable and non-modifiable risk factors such as the weather versus your clothing. Non-modifiable risk factors are out of your control — such as the rain or burning summer sun — something you just must accept. These include your genetics and your age. Modifiable risk factors, on the other hand, are like your choice of clothing — a raincoat or broad-brimmed hat — you can adjust these to better deal with the day's weather, such as improving your diet or increasing your physical activity to influence your health outcomes.

According to Alzheimer's Disease International's (ADI) 2024 Lancet commission report, 14 modifiable risk factors account for around 45 percent of worldwide dementias.

TIP

Here are the Lancet Commission's recommendations based on the 14 modifiable risk factors:

>> Limited education in early life significantly raises risk, so prioritize quality schooling.

>> Address untreated hearing loss with hearing aids to reduce risk.

>> Managing LDL cholesterol is crucial for lowering risk.

>> Depression often comes before dementia; managing it early is vital.

>> Head injuries from accidents or sports elevate risk, so focus on prevention.

>> Regular physical activity supports heart health, weight management, and mental well-being.

>> Type 2 diabetes increases risk, though the role of medication remains unclear.

>> Smoking raises risk, but quitting at any age still helps.

>> Treat midlife hypertension to lower risk.

>> Midlife obesity is linked to dementia, so focus on diet and exercise.

>> Excessive alcohol consumption (more than 21 units per week) adds to risk.

>> Staying socially connected helps, though specific activities aren't yet proven to protect.

>> Air pollution worsens risk, so advocate for better air quality.

>> Untreated vision loss contributes to 2 percent of dementia cases, so prioritize eye care in later life.

REMEMBER

Prevention is our best defense, and the evidence on dementia and AD risk-reduction is conclusive. People who lead mentally, socially, and physically active lifestyles are less likely to develop age-related brain disorders. If you're following this plan as closely as possible while receiving the benefits of modern-day health-care, you have a good opportunity of adding not only years to your life, but also life to your years!

3

Beyond Aging: Other Factors That Impact Brain Health

Learn how eating healthy food supports your brain, from boosting mood to protecting against aging.

Increase physical activity to boost brain health and explore ways to integrate movement into your daily life.

Discover why sleep is your brain's best tool for memory, mood, and long-term health.

Build strong social connections to keep your brain healthy and resilient.

Challenge your mind to build cognitive reserve and protect against aging.

IN THIS CHAPTER

» Exploring sex and gender in the brain

» Understanding male and female sex hormones

» Sex differences in brain structure and function

» Addressing brain health risk in men

» Knowing the neurobiology of puberty, pregnancy, and menopause

Chapter **9**

Understanding the Interplay of Sex and Gender in Brain Health

In this chapter, I cover how sex and gender influence brain health across the lifespan. This chapter guides you through tricky conversations concerning biological sex and experiences of gender from a neuroscience perspective. You look at the special issues men confront regarding brain health. And explore how puberty, pregnancy, and perimenopause alter brain function in biological women.

Full disclosure: This isn't my first rodeo; I've written two books about women's brain health. One of the elements I learned from that research was that the relationship between nature (neurobiology) and nurture (life experiences) is far from obvious. A complicated combination of hormones, genes, and experiences constantly shapes everyone's brain.

TECHNICAL STUFF

In this chapter, I'll distinguish between "sex" (biological differences like chromosomes and anatomy) and "gender" (roles, behaviors, and expectations based on societal norms). I also acknowledge that not everyone identifies strictly as male or female, and gender may not always align with biological sex. Many people identify as non-binary or another gender. My goal is to clearly discuss brain health while recognizing diverse identities and experiences.

Approaching Sex and Gender Differences in the Brain

The conversation over the extent to which male and female brains differ has persisted for decades. Part of the debate about sex differences is how much your biological sex determines the sex of your brain — and if you do indeed have a "brain sex," whether that has consequences for all thoughts, feelings, behaviors, aptitudes, and personality.

How different are the differences?

The basic question asked is whether a man's brain is "male" (or from Mars and colored blue!) and a woman's brain is "female" (from Venus and pink!) and whether you can determine someone's sex by looking at their brain or brain scan.

Asking whether there are male brains and female brains is like asking whether red meat is good for you — neuroscientists can't seem to agree! Some headlines claim brain differences between men and women are so profound they may as well be separate species (or even aliens from different planets!). Other headlines announce no differences at all. Even now, new findings about differences continue to emerge.

Understanding sex differences and sexual dimorphism

The terms "sex differences" and "sexual dimorphism" are often used interchangeably in discussions about biological sex, gender, and neurobiology, but they have distinct meanings in biology.

>> **Sex differences:** These are differences between males and females in anatomy, physiology, or behavior that may come about via any number of genetic, hormonal, developmental, or environmental factors. For example, Multiple Sclerosis (MS) is a neurological disorder that shows a sex difference whereby women are about two to three times more likely to get MS than men.

>> **Sexual dimorphism:** This term refers to distinct physical differences between the sexes of a species beyond just their reproductive organs. Peacocks are a colorful example of sexual dimorphism: Only the male sports a large flamboyant green and blue tail, whereas peahens are brown and have a basic tail dragging along behind them.

Sometimes, debate arises because people are trying to claim that humans' brains are *sexually dimorphic* (as distinct as male and female genitals or peacock's tails) instead of understanding there are small, subtle *sex differences* (more like the difference between male and female hearts, lungs or kidneys).

Taking a bio-psycho-social approach to sex differences

A *bio-psycho-social approach* to sex and gender differences in the brain considers how biological factors (sex) and environmental influences (gender) converge to shape brain development and function. Hormones and genes are crucial in setting up brain structure during development, and the brain continues to adapt in response to life stages like puberty and, in females, pregnancy and menopause. The brain is also shaped by life experiences, such as educational opportunities and societal roles

Understanding WEIRD brains

REMEMBER

In the discussion on aging in Chapter 8, I touch on the importance of study design in understanding how fluid and crystallized mental abilities change throughout life. Similarly, research into sex differences often overlooks the impact of a person's age and life stage. Many studies focus on *WEIRD* people only — ones from Western, Educated, Industrialized, Rich, and Democratic societies. WEIRD people don't fully represent human diversity (and often they're young male college students)! Being WEIRD can skew data and affect how we understand sex differences in the brain.

TIP

Here's one way to think about it. Say you're comparing the brain structure and function of a 19-year-old male lacrosse-playing Harvard freshman, a 31-year-old pregnant woman living in rural India, a 55-year-old male lawyer living in Portugal, and a 93-year-old woman with dementia living in a nursing home in New Zealand. MRIs of their brains won't provide a clear or accurate view of sex differences. Their life experiences and current contexts are vastly different, making comparisons almost laughable!

Gender inequality changes brain structure

A 2023 study published in the journal PNAS may illustrate how gendered experiences influence brain development. The researchers analyzed 7,876 MRI scans from 29 countries to show how gender inequality affected brain structure in women. In countries with low gender equality (for example, India, Brazil, and Turkey), women tended to have thinner cortices in the right hemisphere than in countries with high gender equality (for example, Finland, Germany, and Sweden). That is, the more inequal or different men's and women's gendered life experiences, the more different their brains.

This insight challenges the simplistic notion that male and female brains are fundamentally different because of biological sex. Instead, it shows that gendered experiences can shape brain structure. The researchers were very careful about drawing direct causation but suggested two possible mechanisms behind the observed structural brain differences linked to lived experiences:

>> **Stress responses:** Girls and women living in gender-unequal societies experience more stress and adversity than boys and men, altering healthy brain development.

>> **Less access to education:** Girls and women in gender-unequal societies often have less access to educational opportunities than boys and men, or what the researchers called "enriched environments," which are essential for healthy brain development.

Examining Hormones and Brain Health Across the Lifespan

Some of the nuanced sex differences in the brain can be partly attributed to varying levels of sex hormone exposure at different ages and life stages. For females, there is a slight increase in estrogen levels post-birth, followed by a significant rise during puberty, fluctuations throughout each menstrual cycle, a sharp increase during pregnancy, and a substantial decrease at menopause. In contrast, males experience increased T levels in utero, at birth, and during puberty, with levels generally remaining stable throughout adulthood. As they age, women undergo a rapid decline in estrogen, while some men experience a smaller but gradual decrease in T levels.

A primer on female sex hormones

Look at the main players in the female hormonal landscape: estrogen and progesterone.

Estrogens and progesterone

Estrogen and progesterone not only regulate reproductive functions but also affect brain health because hormone receptors are present in the brain.

>> **Estrogen** is the primary female sex hormone produced mainly in the ovaries. It's responsible for developing female secondary sexual characteristics, such as breast development during puberty. It plays a crucial role in regulating the menstrual cycle via the hypothalamic pituitary ovarian (HPO) axis. Beyond its reproductive functions, estrogen helps maintain healthy bones and supports skin and joint health, cardiovascular function, and, of course, brain health.

>> **Progesterone,** another key female hormone, is produced in the ovaries, after ovulation. Its main role is to prepare the uterus for a potential pregnancy by thickening the uterine lining. Progesterone also maintains this lining during pregnancy, preventing muscle contractions that could lead to early labor. Additionally, it helps regulate the menstrual cycle (via the HPO axis) and supports the early stages of pregnancy.

Estrogen is a group of hormones: estradiol, estrone, and estriol. Estradiol is the main estrogen, crucial for sexual development and the menstrual cycle. Estrone is prominent after menopause, while estriol is produced by the placenta during pregnancy.

Ovarian hormones and the brain

Because the female brain contains estrogen and progesterone receptors, ovarian hormones can influence brain structure and function. There aren't as many receptors for progesterone in the brain as there are for estrogens, so it's been overlooked by research. But it's starting to become clearer that it too can regulate thinking, mood, and neuroplasticity and may even play a role in recovery from brain injury.

While it's common for men to seek out their T levels, its less common to measure ovarian hormone levels in women as they move about so much over the course of a month.

Using female sex hormones as a scapegoat

Sadly, female sex hormones, particularly estrogen, are used as a convenient scapegoat for mood disorders, psychiatric issues, and cognitive dysfunctions in women, especially during critical life stages such as puberty, pregnancy, and menopause.

WARNING

Phrases such as "she's just being hormonal" are often used to dismissively attribute any cognitive or emotional issue a woman is experiencing to ovarian hormones. This perspective assumes that the mere presence of estrogen is synonymous with dysfunction and decline. However, current research challenges this notion, showing that for some women, it's fluctuations in hormone levels that can lead to problems with mood or emotional regulation.

A primer on male sex hormones

Testosterone (T) is the star sex hormone for males, but it's not just about strong bones, big muscles, and masculinity. T plays a role in brain health, influencing neural networks responsible for motivation, attention, and sexual behaviors. High T levels are associated with enhanced spatial skills but can also lead to increased aggression. Conversely, in some men, low T is linked to cognitive and emotional symptoms such as depression, fatigue, and irritability.

T across the lifespan

T is a critical hormone for male health, peaking in the late teens (around age 19) at an average level of 15.4 nmol/L (nanomoles per liter, a unit of concentration) and typically decreasing to about 13.0 nmol/L by age 40. After 40, there's considerable variation in T levels among men, some men's levels remain relatively stable and others drop but only by around one percent per year. Thus, there is no "andropause" or male equivalent to menopause.

LOWER T LEVELS IN FATHERS?

Since 1983, the Philippines' Cebu Longitudinal Health and Nutrition Survey has monitored hundreds of boys and men, tracking how T levels change as men become fathers. After fatherhood, high-T males, who are typically more successful in "mating and dating," show remarkable drops in T levels. The study's biological anthropologist, Lee Gettler, says this decline allows males to focus on raising their children rather than finding new partners. Fathers' T levels are dose-dependent: The more they parent, the lower their T!

The role of T in the male brain

T is produced in the testes and released into the bloodstream and being a steroid hormone, it easily crosses the blood-brain barrier into the brain. Recall in Chapter 6, I discussed how it influences the "masculinization" of the male brain as early as in utero.

T exerts its effects via androgen receptors scattered through the male brain. Androgen receptors lock onto both T and its metabolites, mediating their effects directly through gene expression or indirectly through signaling pathways that influence neuronal activity and synaptic plasticity. High concentrations of androgen receptors are found in the hypothalamus (involved in regulating sexual behaviors), amygdala, hippocampus, and PFC.

T is also metabolized in the brain via a pathway that involves the enzyme 5-alpha-reductase, which converts T into dihydroT (DHT). DHT is a more potent androgen than T.

And in news that usually comes as a surprise to most people, in the brain, T is also metabolized by an enzyme called aromatase into estradiol (Mother Nature was having a good laugh here!). High concentrations of aromatase and estradiol receptors are found in regions similar to androgen receptors (such as, the hypothalamus, amygdala, hippocampus, and PFC).

T replacement (TRT) for when levels are low

T replacement therapy (TRT) is the primary treatment for men with hypogonadism — insufficient T production due to problems with their testicles (such as cancer) or their pituitary gland. Hypogonadism can affect men's fertility, sexual function (both their libido and ability to get an erection), muscle strength, and emotional well-being. TRT stabilizes T levels, but requires comprehensive clinical evaluation and ongoing monitoring, including of prostate health.

REMEMBER

While T levels do fall slightly with age — about one percent per year after your 40s — not all symptoms of aging are caused by loss of hormones, and not all men are appropriate candidates for TRT.

T, mood, and "roid rage"

You may well be aware many men who use TRT haven't be diagnosed with hypogonadism. Some men use it to combat the natural age-related fall in T. Others are motivated by a desire to beef up muscle mass, gain strength, or improve their libido. This is sometimes characterized by the stereotype of "gym bros" with "roid rage" — an outburst of anger, aggression, or violence attributed to the use of anabolic steroids. In animal studies, T is directly associated with more aggressive behavior, but humans are more complex (and have a pre-frontal cortex than can hopefully modify mood!). The link between T levels and TRT and violent behavior is complex and likely affected by a wide range of social, economic, and genetic variables.

Some reported risks of TRT misuse include sleep apnea, acne, prostate enlargement, and increased risk of cardiovascular disease. Clinicians generally advise against the widespread use of TRT in younger men who do not have clear clinical evidence of hypogonadism.

Comparable to studies on estrogen, mood disorders are more closely associated with dramatic changes in T levels than with persistently low levels. While low T levels are associated with depressive disorders in certain men, high levels of T can increase the incidence of depression. Notwithstanding these contradictory results, there is little data to suggest that men with major depressive illness are usually affected by low T levels.

Sex differences and neurodevelopmental disorders

When it comes to neurodevelopmental disorders such as autism and ADHD, boys are diagnosed more frequently than girls, especially before puberty. For example, for every five cases of ADHD, four will be diagnosed in boys. Similar statistics are reported for autism. These sex differences can be due to a mix of biological, social, and diagnostic factors.

>> Biologically, boys may be more susceptible to these disorders due to genetic and hormonal differences. And one theory suggests the male placenta is more vulnerable to the passage of virus or stress hormones, rendered the male fetus suspectable during crucial prenatal brain development.

>> Socially, girls may develop different coping mechanisms that help mask symptoms, leading to underdiagnosis.

>> Historically, diagnostic criteria looked at how boys typically behaved and thus missed how they appear in girls (who are often socialized to conform). Fitting with this notion is the growing trend of middle-aged women being diagnosed with ADHD, highlighting this phenomenon of "masking." Many women develop strategies to cope with their symptoms, often going unnoticed or misdiagnosed for years.

Sex differences and mood disorders

Statistics vary slightly, but for every three cases of depression, two are in women, a statistic mirrored in anxiety disorders. During childhood and early puberty, anxiety and depression rates are similar between boys and girls. However, from puberty onward, a gender gap emerges and persists into old age.

Men suffer from depression too, but they're slightly more likely to be diagnosed with what are called "externalizing disorders" such as drug and alcohol abuse, violence, or aggression. Girls and women tend to develop what are called "internalizing" disorders and often for the first time around adolescence. These include panic disorder, phobias, social anxiety disorder, obsessive-compulsive disorder and eating disorders, and post-traumatic stress disorder (PTSD). Once again, it is worth reminding you these are average differences and there is plenty of overlap between the sexes.

The question of why women are more vulnerable to depression and anxiety is complex, involving multiple interacting biological sex and gender differences and include:

>> Genetic and hormonal differences

>> Reproductive life events or stages especially the menstrual cycle, pregnancy, and menopause

>> A dampened stress response in women

>> Lower self-esteem and a higher tendency for body shame and rumination

>> Higher rates of experienced violence and childhood sexual abuse

>> Lack of gender equality and discrimination

Sex differences and brain aging

As you age, your brain undergoes various changes. I cover the aging brain in detail in Chapter 8 if you want to head there for a review. Sometimes these changes can show up differently between men and women.

>> **Alzheimer's Disease (AD):** Predominantly affects women due to longer lifespans and factors such as hormonal changes post-menopause, combined with socio-economic factors such as historically lower educational and employment opportunities.

- >> **Parkinson's Disease (PD):** More common in men, but women experience higher mortality and faster progression, potentially due to environmental, genetic, or hormonal differences.

- >> **Brain tumors:** Sex differences manifest with men more likely to develop aggressive glioblastomas, and women more prone to certain benign meningiomas, influenced by hormonal factors.

- >> **Motor neuron diseases (ALS):** Men are more likely to develop ALS, but the incidence rate equalizes after age 70, indicating that age-related factors may outweigh hormonal influences in older adults.

REMEMBER

Keep in mind that a different combination of biological, psychological, and environmental factors and life experiences influences sex differences in risk factors for various neurological conditions. However, to date, treatments are usually the same for both men and women. Similarly, when it comes to methods for lowering your risk, advice is broadly the same for both men and women.

Addressing Brain Health in Men

In this section, you explore brain health issues from the perspective of the male lifespan. As I guide you through this section on men's brain health, you see that men face distinct challenges and risks that can affect their mental and neurological well-being.

REMEMBER

When you consider occupational risks and their effects on men's brain health, you'll find significant differences between the sexes, particularly outside Western, Educated, Industrialized, Rich, and Democratic (WEIRD) societies. These disparities are not mentioned to reinforce gender stereotypes but to recognize that men and women often occupy different roles especially in the developing world, which exposes them to varying risks.

Hormonal influences

Testosterone (T) plays a crucial role in shaping the male brain, influencing everything from mood regulation to cognitive function. In young men, healthy T levels are associated with good mental health, sharp cognitive abilities, and robust physical health. However, as men age, T levels naturally decline slightly. Sometimes, this phase is called andropause, but unlike the abrupt hormonal changes of women's menopause, "andropause" resembles a very gradual tapering off, not a steep drop-off.

That said, this decline can impact mood, leading to symptoms such as irritability and depression, and affect cognitive functions such as memory and concentration. Older men may choose to monitor their hormone levels through regular check-ups with a family doctor. For those experiencing symptoms of hypogonadism, healthcare providers may discuss options such as lifestyle changes (healthy food, exercise, sleep, and stress reduction) or TRT.

Risk factors for neurological disorders

Compared to women, men are at a higher risk for certain neurological disorders such as Parkinson's disease (PD) and schizophrenia. Parkinson's disease, for example, tends to be more prevalent in men, possibly due to a combination of genetic, environmental, and lifestyle factors. Men (especially when they're young) are more likely to engage in high-risk behaviors, such as excessive alcohol consumption, vaping, smoking, and taking cannabis, none of which tip the scales towards better brain health.

From heart health to brain health

As you age, you experience changes in cognitive function, which can range from those tip-of-the-tongue moments to (but hopefully not!) more serious issues such as dementia. Interestingly, men's cognitive decline is closely linked to cardiovascular health. In fact, men are more likely to be diagnosed with fronto-temporal vascular dementia than women (this is the form that Bruce Willis has recently revealed he's suffering with).

TIP

So, gentlemen, the more you do to take care of your heart, the better for your brain health. And it's never too soon or too late to start.

Mental health: "Man up" is not the answer!

Mental health problems in men can often go under-recognized and under-treated. This can have devastating consequences.

Mental health symptoms sometimes manifest differently in men. They may feel angry, irritable, drink too much, or behave recklessly, rather than the typical stereotypical sadness or withdrawal. And no matter where in the world you live, there's still stigma associated with men seeking help for mental health issues, which can prevent many from accessing the support they need.

TIP

It's vital to watch out for your friends and maintain relationships. Men's health organizations the world over promote the mental health benefits of community and relationships, such as sports teams, social organizations, and the like.

SUICIDE RATES AMONG MEN

The Australian Bureau of Statistics annually reports on suicide rates, and the 2022 figures highlight a concerning trend: about 75 percent of suicides were men. Specifically, 2,455 men, translating to 18.8 per 100,000 population, tragically ended their lives compared to 794 women, or 5.9 per 100,000. Men over 85 years old, despite representing the smallest demographic at 2.9 percent, had the highest suicide rates among their age group. Meanwhile, men aged 45-49 showed the highest rates among those under 80 years old, making up 10.7 percent of male suicides. These statistics underscore the profound challenges faced by men, particularly as they age.

Occupational hazards and brain health

Compared to women, men are more likely to work in places that put their brain health at risk, such as construction sites, factories, or military settings. These occupations can expose men to the risks of falls, toxin exposure, and high levels of stress or potential for trauma.

It's easy to roll your eyes at occupational health and safety measures, but proper safety equipment, regular health screenings, and workplace mental health support can mitigate these risks. Governments, employers, and employees alike must be proactive in creating safer work environments that prioritize men's physical and mental health.

Delving into Brain Health in Women

In this section, you explore brain health issues from the perspective of women's reproductive health throughout the lifespan. I address specific brain health topics, including the menstrual cycle, hormonal contraceptives, pregnancy, and menopause. Puberty is discussed in detail in Chapter 7.

Charting the menstrual cycle: How estrogen rewires the brain

Estrogen is quite the multitasker in the female brain regulating the menstrual cycle and playing a crucial role in brain plasticity. Estrogen helps regulate the formation and function of dendritic spines — those tiny, bud-like structures on dendrites essential for synapses sending and receiving information. This is especially apparent in the hippocampus. However, the amygdala, as well as the basal ganglia and PFC, appear to be particularly sensitive to the effects of ovarian hormones.

What this means more broadly for cognition across the menstrual cycle is an open question. Most brain imaging studies find no consistent alterations in cognitive brain networks such as decision–making, attention, or planning in healthy women during various phases of the menstrual cycle. This is good news and proves women can work cognitively demanding jobs throughout their reproductive years and beyond!

However, many women say hormonal changes during their menstrual cycle, especially in the luteal phase, can affect how they feel.

PMS and PMDD: Vulnerability to hormonal change

Premenstrual Syndrome (PMS) and Premenstrual Dysphoric Disorder (PMDD) highlight how sensitive some female brains are to hormonal fluctuations.

>> PMS causes mood swings, irritability, and physical symptoms and is tightly linked to the last week of the luteal phase of the menstrual cycle when sex hormone levels drop. Rates for PMS are hard to pin down and vary wildly from country by country. One meta-analysis collated reported rates of PMS by country and found rates varied by country from ten percent to 90 percent!

>> PMDD is a more severe form of PMS, impacting about five percent of women. To be diagnosed with PMDD, women must have five of eleven symptoms, including mood swings, irritation, anxiety, or depression, to be diagnosed with PMDD.

There are four theories for what causes PMDD (and they're probably all partly responsible):

>> Abnormal response to physiological fluctuations of ovarian hormones in brain regions associated with emotional and cognitive processing during the luteal phase of the menstrual cycle

>> Altered sensitivity of GABA A receptors to allopregnanolone (a metabolite of progesterone)

>> Modifications in the function of the serotoninergic system

>> Genetic factors

Investigating the brain health impacts of hormonal contraceptives

Hormonal contraceptives (the pill) work by suppressing your natural levels of ovarian hormones and simultaneously elevating levels of synthetic hormones for very short bursts every day (the half-life of synthetic hormones is only a few hours, which is why you need to take the pill daily). By doing this, they significantly alter the hormonal environment in many women, often for years at a time. Many women take the pill for years and experience no side effects apart from unwanted pregnancy. Other women have sides effects related to mood.

Does the pill cause depression?

If you spend any time online listening to conversations about women's reproductive health, you have likely heard about the potential link between hormonal contraceptives (the pill) and depression.

TECHNICAL STUFF

One study of over one million Danish women found a 23-percent increased relative risk of being prescribed antidepressants for those on the pill, with teenagers showing an 80-percent increase. While media exaggerated the findings, the actual rise in absolute risk was small: out of 100 women, 5 not on the pill and 9 on the pill may need antidepressants. The increased risk was mainly for teenagers, suggesting a link between hormonal contraceptives and adolescent brain development.

Cognitive benefits and risks of the pill

Studies find the pill does not dramatically enhance or impair cognitive function but does lead to nuanced changes (some cognitive skills are improved slightly, others dampened, but it depends on which pill formulation you take, how long you've been using it, and how old you are!). Part of the confusion has been researchers have focused so intently on estrogen they've overlooked the role of progestins (synthetic progesterone) and their metabolites. So, watch this space!

WARNING

Given the benefits of hormonal contraceptives, such as highly effective birth control and reduced cancer risk, it's important to weigh benefits against the potential risks such as increased depression or in blood clots in some women.

Assessing brain changes during pregnancy and motherhood

About 85 percent of women become mothers. Almost all of them would agree that pregnancy and motherhood change them in significant ways physically, mentally, socially, and spiritually. Neuroscientists increasingly recognize pregnancy and parenting as major neurological transitions. Just as women's bodies and lifestyles undergo profound and significant changes, so too do their brains.

Pregnancy prepares the mind for motherhood

The first brain imaging research published in *Nature Neuroscience* in 2017 showed that pregnant women's brains experience significant structural reorganization in cortical networks responsible for social cognition — reading the thoughts, feelings, and needs of others. The mother's brain becomes very plastic and extremely sensitive to and ready to respond to social cues from an infant's cries, cuteness, and smell. (It's a good thing babies are cute as they cry, yet we can't resist cuddling them!)

The "unparalleled estrogen exposure" that occurs in the third trimester causes dramatic neuroplasticity and enhanced flexibility, efficiency, and responsiveness. These changes likely contribute to the psychological processes that help a pregnant woman in getting ready for the arrival of her baby.

Baby brain: Cognitive decline or stereotype?

Around four out of five women report experiencing so-called "baby brain," describing feelings of absent-mindedness or forgetfulness during their pregnancy and early motherhood. However, cognitive testing often shows subtle or mixed results.

In the animal kingdom, new mothers outperform their childless counterparts in problem-solving, learning, stress management, and resilience. And human moms show similar strengths. Some studies suggest a cognitive boost during late pregnancy.

I think the concept of "baby brain" may benefit from a more positive framing. Maternal brain neuroscientists suggest viewing this period as one of cognitive reorganization and adaptation, where the brain is not deteriorating or in deficit but rather becoming more efficient, flexible, and primed for learning skills vital to parenting.

Postnatal depression and anxiety

Statistics typically state at least one in every five women (and one in ten new dads) experience anxiety, depression, or both during pregnancy or following birth (the all-encompassing term I use is "perinatal mood and anxiety disorders") with rates of depression hitting a life-time high after giving birth.

TIP

Many new parents face common challenges, yet often they don't ask for help early, and hence the impact can build up over time, placing everyone under greater stress. Some women brush issues off as "just the baby blues," (and haven't we all felt the pressure to live up to expectations of "coping" versus openly discussing disappointment, frustration, anger, sadness).

Symptoms of postnatal anxiety include changes in:

>> Mood including, worry, feeling nervous, on edge, stressed, panicky, feelings of impending doom, excessive fears, catastrophizing, and obsessive, compulsive, or intrusive thoughts

>> Behavior including panic attacks, inability to sleep or eat, feeling dizzy, urges to self-harm, or developing obsessive or compulsive behaviors

>> Relationships including avoiding people or places that may trigger anxiety or a panic attack, withdrawing from friends and family, worry about telling your postnatal care team what's happening

Symptoms of postnatal depression include changes in:

>> Mood, including feeling sad, low, hopeless, inadequate, like a failure, frequent crying, brain fog, feeling disconnected from your baby or loved ones, anger or thoughts of death or suicide

>> Behavior, including lack of energy or motivation, problems sleeping or eating, urges to self-harm

>> Relationships, including withdrawing from friends and family, arguments, little or no interest in daily activities that usually bring joy

The main risk factors for developing PND and anxiety include:

>> Previous history of depression or mental health disorders

>> Lack of support from family, friends, or community

>> Relationship issues including significant stress in the relationship with a partner

>> Stressful life events such as financial problems or the death of a loved one

>> Complications in pregnancy or childbirth, including a difficult delivery or premature birth

>> Baby's health issues, especially if the newborn has a chronic illness or special needs

>> Hormonal changes (especially plummeting estradiol levels) that naturally occur during and after pregnancy

>> Sleep deprivation and adjusting to the new role and responsibilities of motherhood

Baby blues or something more serious?

WARNING

This *Dummies* book is not the place to figure out whether or not you crossed the line from "baby blues" or ambivalence or feeling tired or stressed or sleep-deprived to a mental health condition that needs treatment.

TIP

As always, the message is "Ask for help and ask early." It is always a good idea to talk to someone (and if you get blown off, talk to someone else). There are also numerous free helplines, drop-in centers, and online resources available in most countries.

Treating PND and anxiety

Depression comes in many shades of blue. A few lifestyle adjustments, such as getting a good night's sleep, exercise, finding a sympathetic ear, or splitting childcare duties, can sometimes help with mild to moderate PND and anxiety symptoms. Sometimes PND, like all depression, is severe and gloomy, with unclear causes. This type of depression requires medical attention. Here's a summary of common treatments:

>> Cognitive behavioral therapy (CBT) is effective for most symptoms.

>> Antidepressants like SSRIs may be used especially for moderate to severe cases.

>> Peer support and group therapy (known in many parts of the world as mother's groups) can offer coping strategies.

>> Exercise, sleep, and nutrition improve mood and overall well-being.

>> Education about PND and counseling can reduce stigma.

>> Mindfulness, yoga, and acupuncture complement other treatments.

Postnatal psychosis

Postnatal psychosis, which affects one to two new mothers in every 1000 in the first couple of months after giving birth, is a far more serious mental health condition that requires emergency psychiatric care. It involves sudden and dramatic changes in a woman's thinking, behavior, mood, sleep patterns, and episodes involving a loss of contact with reality and unusual or erratic behavior. In Australia and New Zealand, women and their babies are often cared for together in specialist mother and baby psychiatric units (often with other family members), and a carefully thought-out plan involving medication, therapy, and social support.

Managing menopause

Menopause marks the end of a women's reproductive life. In short, menopause happens because you run out of eggs and is marked by cessation of your period. In Australia, the average age for natural menopause is 51, but it can occur earlier or later. There's a wide age-range in women who have their last period (anywhere between 40 to 58, 51 years is just the average). We now understand that the years leading up to the last period, known as perimenopause, are also a time of considerable change.

Even though menopause is mostly thought of as the end of your reproductive life, most of the symptoms are neurological in origin!

Signs, symptoms, and definitions

Here are some common symptoms of perimenopause (the years leading up to menopause) and menopause include:

>> Hot flushes, night sweats, or feeling hot or cold

>> Vaginal changes such as dryness and painful intercourse

>> Mood swings, which may include low mood, anxiety, or irritability

>> Cognitive issues, often called "brain fog"

>> Joint or muscle aches, pains, and crawling or itchy skin

>> Headaches and tiredness

>> Lowered libido

There's a silver lining, too! As your hormones stabilize, many women experience a significant boost in their well-being. You may feel more serene, enjoying consistently better moods, and experiencing a richer, more fulfilling quality of life in your 50s and 60s.

Brain changes during menopause

The first brain-imaging study showing how women's brains change during menopause was published by Lisa Mosconi and her colleagues in 2021 (better late than never, I suppose!).

Mosconi scanned the brains of 161 women, including 30 pre-menopausal, 57 peri-menopausal, and 74 post-menopausal participants. Here's a summary of the findings on menopausal brain changes as seen with brain imaging:

>> **Grey matter volume:** Slight decrease during perimenopause with a subsequent increase post-menopause (you could say grey matter volume bounced back!)

>> **White matter organization:** Extensive changes in white matter volume but post-menopausal women show more efficient organization.

>> **Glucose metabolism:** Decrease in glucose metabolism, increased blood flow and ATP production.

>> **Amyloid beta deposition:** Increased deposition in post-menopausal women, especially with APOE-4 allele, raising Alzheimer's risk.

These brain imaging findings illustrated that menopause is a neurological transition involving brain adaptation and plasticity.

The neurobiology of hot flashes and night sweats

Hot flashes are felt by approximately 80 percent of women in the years preceding their final period and often for years afterwards.

TIP

Hot flashes start in your brain, specifically the hypothalamus, which acts like a neural thermostat. It maintains your body temperature around 37°C or 98.6°F by setting thresholds for heat and cold. If you're too hot, it triggers sweating and vasodilation; if too cold, shivering occurs. And your behaviors, such as throwing on a hoodie or throwing off your bedding, also help regulate your temperature.

During perimenopause, these thresholds adjust — making you much more sensitive to temperature changes. A slight rise in core temperature can cause your hypothalamus to overreact, panic even, resulting in hot flashes: You go red, sweat, and feel a burst of adrenaline designed to wake you up and get you moving somewhere cooler. Because the hypothalamic thermostat thresholds are set by estrogen levels, treatments such as hormone replacement therapy (HRT) or menopause hormone therapy (MHT) are effective in reducing hot flashes and improving sleep disturbed by night sweats.

TECHNICAL
STUFF

One drug on the market, fezolinetant, helps treat hot flashes by acting directly on the hypothalamic neural thermostat. It blocks neurokinin-3 receptors in the brain, reducing the activity of KNDy (pronounced candy) neurons responsible for regulating body temperature. In a sense, the drug reinstates the body's internal temperature control.

Brain fog: Not mild cognitive decline

As women transition through menopause, memory concerns are quite common. They're often described colloquially as brain fog.

TIP

A useful definition of *brain fog* is proposed by women's cognitive health researcher Pauline Maki is:

> The constellation of cognitive symptoms experienced by women around the menopause, which most frequently manifest in memory and attention difficulties and involve such symptoms as difficulty encoding and recalling words, names, stories or numbers, difficulty maintaining a train of thought, distractibility, forgetting intentions (reason for coming into a specific room), and difficulty switching between tasks.

Firstly, I assure you, midlife brain fog does not spell inevitable cognitive decline into dementia! Brain fog is a commonly reported (peri)menopause symptom versus an early sign of AD (which remains rare at this age). Compared to young healthy fertile women, some menopausal women perform worse on cognitive tests (especially tasks of verbal memory and fluency). But often they recover post-menopause. Here are various potential causes of brain fog and memory loss during menopause:

» **Hormonal fluctuations:** Menopausal symptoms mainly relate to hormonal fluctuations, not necessarily indicating early mild cognitive impairment (MCI) or Alzheimer's disease (AD), which are uncommon at this stage.

» **Loss of estrogen:** Directly alters synaptic plasticity in cognitive regions.

» **Metabolic changes:** Impair cognitive functions by influencing glucose metabolism and bioenergetics in the brain.

» **Sleep disturbance:** Night sweats and hot flashes can disrupt sleep, adversely affecting mood and cognitive clarity, particularly verbal learning and memory.

» **Stress:** Stress from parenting, caregiving, work, and relationships in the late 40s and 50s can worsen cognitive difficulties.

» **Mood disorders:** Stress and mood disorders during this period can exacerbate memory issues and concentration problems.

Different women experience different trajectories

Like other major life changes, menopause encompasses a wide range of experiences that are very different for each woman. Some enter their goddess phase (which I plan to do), whereas others feel this phase of life is the last taboo and that there is a stigma talking about the "climacteric."

Consider the different cognitive profiles that appear during this important time by looking at specific data from a small but insightful study. The 2021 study by Maki and colleagues tracked 117 perimenopausal women, each undergoing detailed cognitive testing twice annually over several years, generating 415 observations. The researchers applied machine learning (AI) techniques and statistical modelling to identify four distinct groups of women.

>> **Cognitively normal:** About 40 percent with no cognitive decline.

>> **Verbal learning and memory challenges:** 20–30 percent struggle with verbal memory, often linked to sleep issues.

>> **Verbal learning and memory strengths:** 20–30 percent show improved verbal memory, with fewer depressive and hot flash symptoms.

>> **Attention and executive function strengths:** 10 percent excel in attention and executive function, reporting fewer sleep problems.

TIP

These four profiles show how memory and "brain fog" experiences can vary among women during menopause, highlighting the individuality of each woman's experience. So, some of you may exhibit cognitive resilience, while others may feel more vulnerable. Both are real.

Menopause and mental health

While menopause and mental health problems are not the same thing, going through perimenopause makes it more likely for women who have never had depression before to experience mood changes and signs of sadness and anxiety. However, the risk goes up for women who've had mood disorders in the past.

To fully understand and deal with these changes, it's important to know what stage of menopause you're in, look at any past or present mental health signs, and think about how your lifestyle and life stresses may affect your mental health.

Hormone therapy and brain health

First, the good news! Fears that replacing estrogen also known as hormone replacement therapy (HRT) *causes* dementia are based on old research.

In the wake of the Women's Health Initiative (WHI) trial in the early 2000s, the perception of HRT was marred by fears of increased risks for serious health issues, including heart attack, cancer, and dementia. Around 50 percent of women around the world stopped! However, follow up studies and new data analysis paint a different picture. We now understand the risks of HRT were overstated. If you start it during a critical window — preferably within ten years after your last period — HRT can offer significant benefits (reducing hot flashes, sleep disturbances, and strengthening bones) without significantly raising the risk of dementia.

But (and this is an important but), this advice on the risk for dementia only stands for women who've had their uterus removed via hysterectomy and can take estrogen-only HRT. For everyone else with an intact uterus, they need a combination of estrogen and progesterone (to avoid certain cancers). As it stands, no menopause society recommends you take HRT to prevent dementia or AD. But of course, in time, that advice may change. Adding to the confusion, the route of hormone administration matters too, so whether you're popping a pill, sticking on a patch, or applying a gel you may tip the risk-benefit scales one way or another.

WARNING

As always, a good women's health doctor can help you weigh the risks and health benefits of taking HRT to treat menopause symptoms. Once they started, most women swear someone will have to peel their hormone patch off their cold dead body!

Identifying hormone-sensitive subgroups

As you read through this section, you may notice some women are particularly sensitive to the hormonal changes that occur during key reproductive events, such as starting the pill, pregnancy, or menopause. Research indicates there's very likely a "hormone-sensitive subgroup" of women who are more vulnerable to mood or cognitive shifts during these life stages.

This sensitivity can be influenced by genes and how hormones interact with the brain. Understanding this variability could pave the way for more tailored approaches to managing and preventing depression and cognitive issues in women likely to be affected. I'm a bit of a fan of thinking about "subgroups" as a useful way to support individual experiences and avoid making too many broad statements.

REMEMBER

Ladies and gentlemen, remember that midlife is when the early warning signs for poor mental or physical health emerge, but it's not too late. Midlife is a unique window of opportunity to invest in futureproofing your brain. It's time to stop, take stock, and invest in a healthy future.

>> Focus on maintaining a healthy weight, staying active, and managing health conditions such as obesity, high blood pressure, and diabetes to support your cognitive health.

>> Take a multi-pronged approach to prevent dementia; addressing multiple risk factors together is more effective.

>> Remember, what's good for your heart is good for your brain. Aim for a blood pressure level of 120/80 mmHg by managing conditions such as high blood pressure, high cholesterol, and diabetes.

>> Stay active with at least 150 minutes of moderate-intensity aerobic exercise every week to lower your dementia risk.

>> Keep socially engaged, especially if you have a history of depression.

>> Avoid excessive alcohol and quit smoking to protect your brain health.

Chapter **10**

Managing Brain Health after Head Injury

E very year, millions of people around the world suffer accidental brain injuries. These can range from minor sports concussions to more severe trauma resulting in coma or death.

This chapter looks at different brain injuries, how they impact people in the long run, and how to effectively manage and prevent them.

Defining Brain Injuries

Brain injuries are dubbed an invisible disability because they can impact how people think, feel, and interact, yet the person may look healthy and well. Brain damage includes several conditions and disorders that temporarily or permanently disrupt healthy brain function. In the brain injury community, the term *brain injury* includes acquired brain injuries (ABI), meaning they come about accidentally, and degenerative brain disorders and diseases such as Alzheimer's disease or brain tumors. But in this chapter, you consider acquired brain injuries. More information on brain tumors and degenerative diseases is in Chapter 4.

Most ABIs happen after birth. There are a lot of different types of brain injuries, such as those that stop the brain from getting blood or oxygen or those that cause a brain injury by hitting the head. But Fetal Alcohol Spectrum Disorder (FASD) caused by mom drinking alcohol when she's pregnant is also considered an ABI.

Causes of brain injuries

People suffer ABI from various events, including:

» Traumatic accident (a fall, car accident, or sporting injury)

» Concussion

» Stroke

» Hypoxia/Anoxia (lack of oxygen)

» Brain tumors

» Infection or disease

» Fetal Alcohol Spectrum Disorder (FASD)

» Assault and domestic violence

Traumatic Brain Injury (TBI)

Traumatic Brain Injury (TBI) occurs when a sudden blow to the head, such as falling and hitting your head, or rapid movement, such as being in a car accident, being violently assaulted, or knocked down in a collision sport, causes damage to the brain. (I use the term "collision" sport after it was once pointed out to me that ballroom dancing is a "contact" sport!)

The severity of a TBI can vary from mild, such as feeling disorientated, to severe, potentially resulting in unconsciousness or coma.

Sometimes, the damage is what's called an *open head injury*, where the skull bone or another object pierces into the brain. Other times, a *closed head injury* occurs when the brain slams around inside the skull, but no bones are broken. Brain tissue damage can be localized (such as damage caused by vascular stroke) or diffuse, impacting widespread brain regions.

Sequence of injury

Diffuse axonal injury happens when the brain is shaken or twisted inside the skull, causing damage to axons (white matter tracts). This type of injury can have serious effects on the brain's function. Here's what typically happens after a closed head trauma:

>> **Immediate impact:** Right after the injury, the brain's axons stretch and tear, disrupting normal brain function.

>> **Secondary injury:** In the hours and days following the trauma, the brain may swell, and blood flow to certain areas may decrease, leading to further damage.

>> **Inflammation:** The body's response to injury includes inflammation, which can worsen the damage by putting more pressure on the brain.

>> **Cell death:** Damaged nerve cells may die off over time, which can lead to loss of brain function in affected areas.

>> **Recovery phase:** The brain begins to heal, but this process can be slow, and some effects may be long-lasting or permanent.

The global burden of TBI

According to the 2022 Lancet Neurology Commission, TBI affects 55 million people globally at any given time, costs over U.S. $400 billion annually, and is a significant cause of death and disability from injuries. TBIs are not just moments in time but are considered chronic health issues, increasing the risk of mental health problems and diseases such as Parkinson's and dementia later in life.

The primary causes of TBI are road accidents and falls. In developing countries, road accidents cause almost three times as many TBIs as falls. On the other hand, in wealthier countries, falls are responsible for twice as many TBIs as road accidents.

Certain groups of people are more at risk of TBI from different causes. For example, young men 20 to 24 are most at risk of TBI from being violently assaulted. Hospitalizations are most common among older adults (over 65) from falls (often due to alcohol use or DIY home repairs). Children and teenagers have the second-highest incidence of hospital admissions for TBI from traffic accidents.

Assessing the severity of TBI

When someone's suspected of having a TBI, they're usually taken to hospital. Here they have a neurological examination, and decisions are made to rule in or out brain surgery to deal with issues such as bleeding, skull fractures, and high intracranial pressure from brain swelling. A variety of imaging tools such as CT scans, MRIs, X-rays, and intracranial pressure monitoring can be used to assess the condition of the brain.

Two reliable measures of TBI severity are the length of any coma and the duration of post-traumatic amnesia. One commonly used tool is the Glasgow Coma Scale (GCS), which grades a person's level of consciousness. The scale runs from three to 15 based on verbal (speaking), motor (movement), and eye-opening reactions to stimuli. A lower GCS score indicates a more severe injury, with scores of three to eight reflecting severe TBI, nine to 12 moderate TBI, and 13 to 15 mild TBI. These measures help doctors determine the extent of brain injury and guide treatment.

Living with TBI

Synapse, Australia's brain injury organization, provides guidance and support to those adjusting to living with TBI. Here are some of their best pieces of advice:

>> **Rehabilitation:** Tailored rehab is essential for recovery and should begin in the hospital and continue at home.

>> **Social support:** Relearning social skills is key for relationships; joining support groups is encouraged.

>> **Health and well-being:** Maintaining physical health aids brain healing through diet, exercise, and following your doctor's advice.

>> **Reintegration:** Returning to school or work can be eased with small adjustments and proper support.

>> **Mental health:** Building routines post-rehab prevents boredom and supports ongoing progress.

Concussions

Concussions are the most prevalent type of TBI, impacting around 42 million people globally each year.

REMEMBER

TBI is a broad term for any brain injury. A *concussion*, on the other hand, is a specific type of mild TBI that happens when a blow or jolt to the head causes temporary changes in brain function. Concussions usually cause symptoms such as headaches, dizziness, and confusion, but these symptoms typically resolve with rest. So, think of a concussion as a mild, temporary form of TBI. While all concussions are TBIs, not all TBIs are concussions. Most people recover quickly from concussions, but brain specialists stress that even minor concussions can have serious consequences, especially if a second occurs before full recovery.

Symptoms of concussion

Concussions symptoms can vary but typically include:

>> Immediate signs such as muscle rigidity, loss of body tone, bladder control, or coordination issues.

>> Ongoing issues such as headaches, nausea, confusion, memory problems, vision changes, and sensitivity to light and sound.

>> Emotional and sleep disturbances, including irritability, sadness, and sleep difficulties.

Diagnosis of concussion is generally based on neurological and cognitive assessments, as the damage is often too subtle for detection via brain scans.

WARNING

Contrary to popular opinion, you do not have to lose consciousness (pass out) to suffer a concussion, and even mild cases should be carefully looked after.

Treatment and recovery

Most people only need rest to recover from a concussion. And it's crucial to resume normal activities gradually.

WARNING

Seek immediate medical attention if symptoms such as worsening headaches, slurred speech, weakness, numbness, or uncoordinated movements appear. Also, watch for severe nausea, vomiting, seizures, loss of consciousness, worsening symptoms, or symptoms that persist beyond ten days.

Some people may experience what's called *post-concussive syndrome*, which includes prolonged symptoms such as memory and concentration issues, mood swings, personality changes, headaches, fatigue, dizziness, insomnia, or excessive drowsiness lasting weeks to months.

Concussions in children

Children, especially boys aged ten to 19, face a higher risk of concussions, mainly from their involvement in collision sports such as ice hockey, rugby, and American football. Sports contribute to a quarter of all concussions, with falls accounting for about half.

Second impact syndrome

With sports concussion, a danger of what's called *second impact syndrome* (SIS) is when a person is concussed for the second time while still healing from a previous concussion, regardless of how minor the injuries are. Here's how it comes about:

>> **Initial concussion:** A first concussion disrupts brain function.

>> **Incomplete recovery:** A second impact occurs before full healing

>> **Rapid brain swelling:** The second injury causes quick cerebral edema.

>> **Neurological deterioration:** The person may quickly lose consciousness.

>> **Potentially fatal outcome:** Without swift intervention, this can lead to brain damage or death.

WARNING

Although rare, SIS can be fatal, which is why it is critical to thoroughly heal from concussion before participating in activities or sports that provide a risk of harm. Young athletes, particularly those in collision sports, are at higher risk because their brains are still developing.

Infections

Infections that lead to swelling in the brain or its protective covering, the *meninges*, can cause significant brain injuries. The two most common infections are encephalitis and meningitis.

Encephalitis

Encephalitis is inflammation of the brain, typically caused by viruses, including herpes and enteroviruses. Symptoms often mimic the flu, such as headaches, fever, light sensitivity, and neck stiffness, but can rapidly escalate to problems with speech, movement, memory, and behavior. Long-term effects can include difficulties with memory, concentration, balance, speech, and language, as well as causing headaches, fatigue, sensory changes, epilepsy, and alterations in mood and behavior.

Meningitis

Meningitis is the inflammation of the meninges and can be initiated by viruses, bacteria, or even physical injuries and certain medications. While viral meningitis may improve with rest, bacterial meningitis is more severe and demands emergency medical treatment. Like encephalitis, it starts with flu-like symptoms that progress to confusion and seizures. The long-term consequences of meningitis can be severe, affecting memory, vision, speech, and balance and may even result in kidney damage.

Vaccinations protect against many bacterial strains responsible for meningitis, which include meningococcal and pneumococcal, among others.

Fetal Alcohol Spectrum Disorder

Fetal Alcohol Spectrum Disorder (FASD) is a collection of conditions caused by exposure to alcohol during pregnancy. It's a sneaky disorder that may not be noticeable at birth but can pop up anytime during childhood or even later in life. This condition affects between two percent to five percent of babies in Australia, and in some marginalized Indigenous communities, the prevalence can soar up to 12 percent.

Alcohol exposure during pregnancy disrupts normal brain development, leading to smaller brain size and altered development in key areas like the frontal lobe, hippocampus, and decreased connectivity between regions.

Signs and symptoms of FASD

FASD can show up as physical signs like a smaller head and distinct facial features or as hidden issues like learning difficulties, cognitive impairments, and behavioral problems. Some children have severe birth defects, such as heart or eye issues, and their brain alterations impact decision-making, learning, memory, and motor control.

Impacts of FASD

The impact of FASD extends beyond childhood health. Without proper support, these children grow up having difficulties in school — both learning and socializing — and later in life securing a job and carry their own risk of substance abuse and mental health problems. It also makes independent living more challenging and can entangle young people in the justice system.

WARNING

The bottom line? There's no safe amount of alcohol when it comes to pregnancy. Steering clear of alcohol during those nine months is the best prevention strategy.

Exploring the Impacts of Brain Injuries

According to Australian research, people who've had a concussion or traumatic brain injury (TBI) may feel different for a long time after the accident. Even though it is now clear that a traumatic brain injury (TBI) can lead to a neurological disease, we still don't know who is most likely to get one or what their outlook may be after an injury.

Longer-term impacts of living with TBI

The impact of a TBI varies widely, depending on where the brain is injured and how severe the injury is. Each person's short- and long-term outcomes are heavily influenced by their emergency care and the ongoing effectiveness of their rehabilitation process.

Cognitive effects

TBI can affect a person's thinking or cognitive skills. Common changes to cognition include the following:

>> Difficulty staying focused affects work, study, and daily tasks.

>> Memory problems like forgetting names, losing thoughts, and misplacing objects are common,.

>> Repetitive behavior or speech may occur due to changes in memory and attention.

>> Problems with organizing and decision-making.

>> Loss of motivation and difficulty starting activities.

Physical effects

TBI can affect a person's physical health. Physical effects may include:

>> Fatigue, sleep issues, and persistent headaches are common and can be disabling.

>> Seizures and sensory processing difficulties affect awareness and perception.

>> Balance problems and dizziness can impair movement.

>> Hearing, visual impairments, and anosmia impact daily functioning.

>> Sexual changes may require open discussions with partners for support.

Behavioral effects

A person with TB might show changes in their behavior, or how they interact with other people or the world around them. Changes to behavior commonly look like:

>> Anger and impulsive behavior is expected due to difficulties with self-regulation.

>> Difficulty viewing situations from others' perspectives can lead to self-centered behavior.

>> Lack of self-awareness makes recognizing and correcting behavior hard.

Psychological effects

TBI can make a person more vulnerable to mental health problems, or less resilient to stress. Some common psychological effects include:

>> Exacerbated stress, anxiety, and panic attacks can impact overall well-being.

>> Increased risk of mental illnesses such as depression and anxiety adds stress for individuals and their families.

>> A higher risk for suicide makes it crucial to recognize warning signs and seek help.

The challenge of predicting recovery

REMEMBER

Predicting recovery after a brain injury is incredibly challenging and often leaves people grappling with enormous uncertainty. There's a saying that the only predictable outcome of TBI is its unpredictability. Synapse Australia says it's important for people and their families to be optimistic but realistic about recovery.

Recovery and learning to live with TBI is a long journey, heavily influenced by an ongoing rehabilitation process, well beyond the initial hospital stay. This rehabilitation and the rehab crew are crucial for the person with TBI adapting to new ways of going about their daily life. Factors such as someone's pre-injury health and age, the severity of their brain injury, their personal resilience, and the support from loved ones, and access to a comprehensive medical team also play determining roles in the recovery process.

Staying healthy after TBI

Recovering from a TBI extends well beyond professional rehabilitation. Key points to support brain health in TBI recovery include:

>> **Mental stimulation:** Use puzzles, games, and books to challenge your brain.

>> **Healthy diet:** Focus on nutrients beneficial for brain health, such as fish, fruits, and vegetables.

>> **Physical exercise:** Engage in activities that raise your heart rate daily.

- >> **Safety measures:** Wear protective gear and take precautions to avoid additional injuries.

- >> **Stress management:** Use relaxation techniques and balance work and recreation.

- >> **Quality sleep:** Prioritize good sleep habits to enhance brain repair and memory.

- >> **Health monitoring:** Regularly check and manage blood pressure, diabetes, and cholesterol levels.

- >> **Avoiding substances:** Limit intake of alcohol and avoid drugs to protect cognitive functions.

A sad result of TBIs: Chronic Traumatic Encephalopathy (CTE)

CTE is a progressive brain disease that develops over years or decades after repeated head trauma, often seen in athletes from sports like rugby, football, and boxing, as well as in military combat and domestic violence survivors. Though symptoms appear long after the injuries, CTE can only be diagnosed after death, and there are no current treatments available.

Signs and symptoms of CTE

CTE develops gradually and can be hard to diagnose during life, showing up as mood changes like depression and anxiety, along with memory loss and confusion. People also experience impulsivity, aggression, and sometimes suicidal thoughts, often years after leaving sports or the military, making it tough to link directly to CTE. After death, CTE is confirmed by examining brain tissue for changes that can't be seen with current imaging. CTE is marked by tau protein buildup, causing memory and emotional issues, but unlike Alzheimer's, tau accumulates around blood vessels in a distinct pattern.

Current controversies surrounding sport concussion and CTE

CTE has become a hotly debated topic, particularly in so-called "collision sports." As awareness of the problem has grown, so too have concerns about the safety of players (including children and elite professionals) taking part in sports with high rates of head trauma, such as tackle rugby, American football, ice hockey, and boxing.

The NFL in the U.S. and World Rugby have been criticized and faced legal action over concussion management, leading to changes in how these sports are regulated and played. Despite progress, resistance from some coaches, fans, and sporting bodies has slowed the implementation of new safety protocols, with some arguing that stricter rules "ruin the game." Still, organizations are now adopting more robust concussion protocols, and age limits for contact sports are being debated as awareness grows about the long-term effects of concussions on young developing brains.

Implementing Concussion Prevention Strategies

The 2022 Lancet Neurology Commission outlined critical areas for preventing TBI, emphasizing tailored strategies for different groups and environments. Prevention efforts must focus on the most common causes of brain injury, which are falls (42%), transportation incidents (29%), and assaults (14%).

Strategies and policies to reduce the harm from TBI

The Lancet Neurology Commission suggests improving road safety to reduce TBIs in developing countries, while wealthier nations focus on preventing falls in older adults. For children, the priority is car safety, traffic education, and protecting young athletes. Global efforts like the WHO's Decade for Action on Road Safety aim to halve traffic deaths by 2030, while in the U.S., the CDC's STEADI initiative focuses on fall prevention for the elderly. In sports, rule changes such as lowering tackle heights in rugby and banning body checking in youth hockey aim to reduce concussions.

Tips to keep your brain safe

TIP

Here are a few ways to significantly reduce the risk of head injuries and maintain a safer environment for yourself and your loved ones.

>> Use a walker or cane to prevent falls if needed.

>> Get regular eye exams and correct vision problems.

>> Monitor medications with your doctor to avoid balance issues.

>> Remove clutter, secure rugs, and improve home lighting to prevent trips.

>> Avoid ladders and get help for tasks requiring climbing.

>> Wear a helmet for cycling, sports, or skiing to reduce head injury risk.

>> Keep your car in good condition and always wear your seatbelt.

IN THIS CHAPTER

» Investigating environmental factors
and their impacts

» Evaluating air and water quality
and toxins

» Adapting to time zones and seasons

» Exploring the impact of
socioeconomic status on brain health

» Comparing urban and rural
environments

Chapter **11**

Wondering at the World: The Environment and Brain Health

ave you ever thought about how the world around you affects your brain health? Maybe you consider the air you breathe (especially if you remember a time when smoking indoors was commonplace!) or the water you drink. But you may be unaware that where you live — big city versus rural farm, proximity to the equator, or even the changing seasons — can influence your brain health.

In this chapter, I show you how the world around you affects your brain and give you some pointers on how to make your environment healthier for your brain.

Investigating Environmental Factors

This chapter explores the surprising connections between the world "out there" and your brain's well-being.

Air quality

One of the most crucial yet often overlooked factors for your health is air quality. The air you breathe significantly impacts your overall health, including your brain. The World Health Organization highlights that addressing air pollution is essential for protecting public health, as it is the second biggest risk factor for noncommunicable diseases globally!

What's in the air?

Air pollution is a complex mix of gases, chemicals, metals, and tiny particles. Fine particles (usually from traffic fumes or burning wood in your home fireplace) are of concern as they're easily inhaled and make their way into your bloodstream. Breathing polluted air for many years or experiencing high levels of air pollution over a short time frame can harm your lungs and heart. The link between air pollution and heart or lung health is well-documented.

Air pollution and dementia risk

A 2022 analysis of 70 studies found a definite link between air pollution and accelerated cognitive decline. While the researchers stopped short of claiming causation, they suggested that the impact may be due to how air pollution affects the cardiovascular system and thus the brain's blood flow. One theory that microscopic pollution particles directly enter the brain, causing inflammation or triggering AD-like plaques, is not currently supported by the data.

TIP

Most weather apps report pollution levels. To reduce your individual risk, if it's a polluted day, stay indoors and avoid exercising outside. And reduce the number of pollutants inside your house (gas cooking, votive candles, and wood fires all add to the mix!).

REMEMBER

Sadly, given that most of the causes of outdoor air pollution are well beyond your individual control, local, national, and regional level decision-makers in fields including energy, transportation, waste management, urban planning, and agriculture must take coordinated action. The best you can do is advocate for a cleaner planet!

Water quality and access

Having access to clean water is among our most fundamental human requirements. But, one in four people worldwide lack access to clean drinking water and about one million people die every year from unsafe water and poor hygiene.

Dehydration can impair cognitive function

Drinking enough water is essential for everyone, no matter your age, but young children, people who are ill or elderly sometimes struggle to drink enough water. Staying hydrated can prevent headaches, confusion, and concentration. As you get older, you may not feel as thirsty, but it's still important to drink regularly.

REMEMBER

Remember, keeping hydrated is key to staying healthy!

Is tap water healthy?

Because all tap water contains trace elements, there is much debate over their significance in dementia risk. In 2024, a review of ten studies took a closer look at the impact of the most common trace elements in tap water — fluoride, calcium, aluminum, and silica. In terms of dementia risk, fluoride played no impact, silica and calcium provided protection, but long-term exposure to aluminum in tap water raised the risk. Interestingly, silica and calcium were shown to diminish AD risk by lowering aluminum absorption. The study emphasizes the importance of understanding how certain substances in drinking water affect our brains, implying that improved water management may help minimize the risk of cognitive decline.

Environmental toxins

A *toxin* is any harmful substance that causes health issues when ingested, inhaled, or absorbed through the skin, and the saying "the dose makes the poison" helps explain toxicity — anything, even water or salt, can be toxic at high doses, while small amounts of harmful substances may not be dangerous.

Depending on where you live, you may be exposed to toxins that can impact brain health. Chronic exposure to certain toxins, such as cigarette smoke, heavy metals (like lead and mercury), pesticides, and industrial chemicals, can lead to neurodevelopmental disorders in children and neurodegenerative diseases in adults, particularly during critical brain development periods like pregnancy and childhood.

Moving Between Time Zones and Seasons

Jetting off to new time zones or navigating through changing seasons puts your brain to the test! There are also some surprising risks and benefits for brain health depending how close to the equator you live!

Globetrotting: The effects of time zone changes

Traveling across different time zones is always a thrill (who doesn't love an international holiday?) but after your long-haul flight is over, it remains challenging for your brain. *Jet lag*, the temporary disruption of your internal clock, can leave you feeling foggy and with difficulty concentrating and sleeping when you need to.

TIP

To ease time zone transitions, adjust your sleep schedule before traveling, reset your clock on the flight, stay hydrated, and get plenty of natural light, especially in the morning, once you arrive.

Seasonal Affective Disorder (SAD)

Seasonal affective disorder (SAD), also known as "fall-winter depression" or the "winter blues," is a type of mood disorder that emerges at the same time of the year making you feel low on energy, craving carbs, and even gaining weight. People with SAD are more likely to live farther from the equator where there are significant seasonal variations in daylight. For example, in Florida, 1 percent of locals experience SAD compared to 15 percent of Canadians!

The lack of sunlight in winter disrupts circadian rhythms, possibly triggering SAD in some people by causing an overproduction of melatonin, the sleep hormone. This excess melatonin leads to increased sleepiness and lethargy, and in those prone to SAD, it interferes with serotonin regulation, affecting mood. For more on melatonin and sleep, see Chapter 14. Skip to Chapter 14 to read more about sleep and melatonin.

TIP

To manage SAD, spending time outside or near a window can boost sunlight exposure, or light therapy may help if natural light isn't available.

Autumn brain: Peak brain performance

Winter leaves some people feeling sad or blue, but surprisingly, other seasons impact your brain and how you think and feel. In 2023, researchers found that autumn is the peak season for brain connectivity, using fMRI scans to track brain activity over the year. This aligns with earlier research showing that cognitive performance also peaks in autumn, influenced by daylight length and temperature changes.

Older adults showed their best cognitive abilities near the fall equinox, with a nearly 30 percent higher chance of cognitive impairment in winter and spring compared to summer and autumn. As the seasons change, so does your brain, so those prone to SAD may want to capitalize on their brain's autumn peak before winter blues set in!

Living Urban versus Rural

Big city living has its pros and cons. It can be stressful, polluted, and busy but offers educational and employment opportunities you can't always access in in the country. City living comes with risk for those with vulnerability to psychiatric issues.

City living as a psychiatric risk factor

WARNING

As outlined in Chapter 4, schizophrenia is a severe psychiatric disorder that affects how a person thinks, feels, and behaves. It can cause symptoms such as hallucinations, delusions, and disorganized thinking, making it one of the most debilitating mental health problems.

Decades of data tracking have shown that living in urban areas increases a person's risk of developing schizophrenia and other psychotic disorders. This connection, known as "urbanicity," puts people living in cities at two to two and half times higher risk compared to people living rurally. Risk also increases for people who move from the country to the city. Factors like social fragmentation, air pollution, and lack of access to green spaces are suggested to contribute to this higher risk.

TIP

Without sounding trite about such a serious condition, one idea is that balancing the benefits of urban living with strategies to reduce stress and increase exposure to nature can help protect your brain health.

Green and blue spaces and mental well-being

No matter where you live, spending time in so-called green and blue spaces — such as parks, gardens, lakes, rivers, or the sea — boosts your mood and improves health.

The way you commute to work can significantly impact your mood. As you'd expect, riding a bicycle, walking, commuting with a friend, or moving near green spaces or water was linked to a more positive mood. On the other hand, noise, crowded footpaths, traffic jams, and busy public transport, as well as commuting alone or driving, tend to make people grumpier and less happy when they arrive at work (no surprise there!).

TIP

That said, if you're not one of the lucky few who have the choice of where to spend your working days try walking or biking, commuting with a friend, or taking scenic routes to make your daily commute healthier and less stressful.

Exploring the Impact of Socioeconomic Status on Brain Health

Socioeconomic status (SES) has a profound impact on children's brain health and how they grow up and function as healthy contributing members of adult society. Children growing up in poverty often face chronic stress, and some researchers look at poverty as a model of toxic stress and adverse childhood experiences (ACEs; we look at this in depth in Chapter 6).

Poverty, stress, and brain development

Healthy brain development in children from low-income households requires access to enriching childhood experiences. Columbia neuroscientist Kimberly Noble's research tested the idea that cash bonuses could provide more opportunities for low-SES families.

In the Baby's First Years study, families receiving $333 per month saw positive impacts on children's social-emotional skills and brain activity compared to those receiving just $20. Even a small cash boost improved children's brain development, language, and cognitive skills. Noble's findings suggest that financial stability plays a crucial role in children's growth and learning. Economic stability and lifting families out of poverty could help children (and their little brains) thrive.

Educational opportunities and brain development

Access to quality education is another critical factor in brain development. Educational opportunities stimulate cognitive growth and help build neural connections. You can read more about healthy childhood development and the role of education in Chapter 6.

4
Keeping Your Brain Healthy

Discover which dietary patterns truly nourish your brain.

Explore how movement powers up your brain health and mental well-being.

Recognize the impact of sleep on mental health and cognition.

Explore social life's role in brain health.

Engage in cognitive challenges to build cognitive reserve, delay dementia onset, and promote overall brain health.

IN THIS CHAPTER

» Thinking about food as more than fuel

» Navigating the contradictions of nutrition science

» Considering the Mediterranean diet

» Linking gut health and brain health

» Answering common questions about nutrition

Chapter **12**

Nourishing Your Brain: Nutrition and Brain Health

In this chapter, you start to understand why the science of nutrition sounds as contradictory as a soap opera! You explore which dietary patterns truly nourish your brain (no need to buy expensive supplements or follow fads), and I guide you through the latest clinical trials on these diets and their remarkable impact on depression, dementia, and other brain disorders. Then I bust some common food myths, and, by the end, you have a clear and practical food prescription for a healthier, happier brain. Get started on this delicious journey!

So What's Food For, Anyway?

Why did we evolve with such complicated digestive systems when other organisms can simply absorb nutrients from their surrounding environment? Read on to find out.

Food is fuel

When it comes to your brain, food is indeed fuel! Your brain consumes 20 percent of your daily energy intake. That's because your neurons are the busiest of your cells.

Food is macronutrients and micronutrients

REMEMBER

Food is more than just fuel. It's also the source of essential building blocks that your body and brain need to grow, repair, and age. Nutrients can be broadly categorized into two groups: macronutrients and micronutrients.

Macronutrients

Macronutrients are the nutrients your body needs in larger amounts. They are the primary sources of energy and the building blocks for various cellular processes.

>> **Carbohydrates** provide glucose, the main energy source for your body and fuel for neurons.

>> **Protein** supplies essential amino acids to build and repair tissues, and synthesize hormones and neurotransmitters.

>> **Fat** provides essential fatty acids, energy, and helps absorb vitamins while forming 60 percent of your brain's structure.

Micronutrients

Micronutrients include vitamins and minerals, needed in microscopic amounts, but are still very important. Vitamins are organic, meaning they're made by living organisms such as plants. Minerals are inorganic, meaning they come from the soil or water. Together vitamins and minerals support a wide range of your physiological and cellular needs. Examples include:

>> Key brain vitamins include B vitamins for energy and neurotransmitter synthesis, Vitamin C for antioxidant protection, and Vitamin E for cell membrane health.

>> Essential minerals like magnesium aid synapse transmission, zinc supports brain function, and iron is vital for oxygen transport and energy metabolism.

Food is an environmental and social signal

Food is about much more than fuel and nutrients. Although you may not have thought about it like this before: Food acts as a powerful signal about the world around you. What you eat reflects the changing seasons, where you live (forest, sea, or mountain top), and the health of the environment you're living in. Food also plays a crucial role in how you gather, share, and connect with other people.

TIP

Sharing an evening meal with your family or a festive banquet with your community is as crucial to your brain health as the vitamins and minerals you consume.

Understanding Nutrition Science and Its Findings

Nutrition science can be a real puzzle, filled with contradictory studies that each have their own flaws and limitations. This messiness is one reason why nutrition advice is so confusing. It's no wonder researchers can't seem to agree on whether tomatoes cause or protect against cancer, or whether alcohol is good or bad for you.

Look at some of the evidence and also why that evidence is so confusing.

Nutrition science is tricky

So, why is nutrition science so tricky? Here are a few key reasons:

>> Running blinded randomized controlled trials (RCTs) for nutrition research are impractical if not impossible.

- Observational studies while common, can't prove cause and effect, only associations.

- Food surveys can be inaccurate because people often misremember or misreport what they ate.

- Conflicts of interest arise when studies are funded by companies with vested interests.

- Food's nutritional content varies by preparation, growth conditions, and sourcing.

- Individual responses to foods vary widely, and nutritional needs change with age, gender, and lifestyle, making personalized diets essential. So there's no one size fits all when it comes to diet.

Studies are contradictory

Often, when it comes to diet, individual studies contradict one another. For example, in a 2013 paper published in the *American Journal of Clinical Nutrition*, academics randomly selected 50 ingredients from recipes in *The Boston Cooking-School Cookbook* and looked at studies on their cancer-causing or cancer-curing potentials. Almost every food had studies claiming both positive *and* negative health effects. (Well, except for olives!).

When you look at this research, it's no wonder that one day tomatoes (or red wine or red meat or blueberries or bacon) are touted as cancer-fighting heroes, and the next day they're banned substances.

My advice is to approach nutrition critically, not take every study or headline at face value, and remember the value of simple, timeless advice like "Eat your fruits and vegetables!"

There's more to diet than individual choices

Diet is influenced by much more than individual choices. The Innocenti Framework, used by the UN to discuss child nutrition, highlights how political, economic, technological, environmental, and cultural forces shape what we eat. This framework reminds us that health is not solely a result of personal responsibility, but also of broader societal factors. For example, the global rise in obesity can't simply be blamed on individuals making "bad lifestyle choices."

Consider the bigger picture when thinking about diet, rather than blaming individuals for poor health outcomes.

Studying the Mediterranean Diet

There is no way to study every macronutrient or vitamin or essential fatty acid in a clinical trial and say that this one is the key to good health. Instead, researchers usually take a broader look at dietary patterns. Even with all the difficulties of nutrition research, it is very important to understand how food affects health, especially because people all over the world eat in very different ways.

The Mediterranean diet (MedDiet) has been widely studied, partly because of its roots in the culinary traditions of countries like Italy, Greece, and Spain, where it has been linked to lower heart disease rates since the 1950s. While some critics argue it's not one-size-fits-all due to regional differences and personal health needs, other diets like the Nordic or Japanese diets also offer health benefits. However, the MedDiet remains one of the best-researched diets, showing many different ways of eating can support good health.

Eating a Mediterranean style diet

The MedDiet, rich in fruits, vegetables, whole grains, legumes, nuts, olive oil, and fish (plus a little red wine), has been linked to numerous health benefits like lower risks of heart disease, diabetes, obesity, dementia, and improved mental health. Its anti-inflammatory, antioxidant properties make it ideal for reducing obesity and, with its plant-based focus, it has a low environmental impact, offering both health and sustainability benefits.

Rather than being a strict optimization protocol, the MedDiet is like a set of guiding principles that influence how you select, prepare, eat, and enjoy food. Here's a quick summary of what you should eat on a Mediterranean-style diet:

>> **Veggies and fruits:** Load up on a variety of colorful vegetables and fruits.

>> **Extra virgin olive oil:** Use this as your main source of fat — it's both tasty and healthy!

>> **Wholegrain breads and cereals:** Think wholegrain goodness such as whole wheat bread and hearty cereals.

>> **Legumes and beans:** Chickpeas, kidney beans, lentils — these are your new best friends.

>> **Nuts and seeds:** Snack on a handful of nuts or sprinkle seeds over your meals.

>> **Fish and seafood:** Treat yourself to fish and seafood regularly.

>> **Herbs and spices:** Flavor your dishes with onion, garlic, and a variety of herbs and spices such as oregano, coriander, and cumin.

Wondering about meat and dairy? No worries! You can definitely include:

>> **Yogurt, cheese, and milk:** Enjoy these in moderation.

>> **Lean proteins:** Chicken, turkey, and eggs are all great choices.

>> **Red meat and sweets:** Keep these to small amounts and occasional treats.

>> **Processed meats and packaged foods:** Try to limit these to rare occasions.

And what about alcohol? If you enjoy a drink, wine (especially red wine) is a traditional part of this diet. Just remember, it's all about moderation and enjoying it with meals.

Taking a Brain Health Approach to Nutrition: The Evidence

You might think we've always known that diet affects brain health, but only recently has strong scientific evidence shown just how crucial a healthy diet is for brain performance, treating depression, and even reducing the risk of Alzheimer's and cognitive decline.

A healthy body is as important as a health brain

Mental illness is a brain disorder? Well, it's tempting to think that's the case and not dig any deeper.

But a powerful new analysis has found poor physical health is a more obvious sign of mental illness than poor brain health. A 2023 *JAMA Psychiatry* paper looked at the health of 85,748 people who'd been diagnosed with psychiatric disorders (for example, schizophrenia, bipolar disorder, depression, and generalized anxiety disorder) and compared them to 87,420 healthy people.

Using a wide range of tests, scans, and assessments, researchers scored the health of different body systems: pulmonary (lung), musculoskeletal, kidney, metabolic, hepatic (liver), brain, cardiovascular (heart and blood vessels), and immune systems. They found that people with psychiatric problems had much lower scores for body health than their healthy peers. The kidneys, liver, immune, and metabolic systems were all hit the hardest (harder in fact than the brain!).

I understand this all may be confronting to think about, but remember you can't separate your mental health from your physical health. If you're dealing with a mental health condition, it's just as important to look after your physical body as it is to look after your mind. And eating a healthy diet is one of the best ways to do that.

Connecting diet and mood disorders

When it comes to protecting yourself from depression, a healthy diet is one of your most useful tools.

Clear evidence MedDiet reduces risk for depression

Eating more plant foods such as vegetables, fruits, legumes, and whole grains, along with lean proteins such as fish, can significantly lower your risk of depression. And, on the flip side, eating lots of ultra-processed factory-made foods and sugary stuff can increase your depression risk.

Studies from around the world consistently show this relationship holds. Meta-analyses (pooled observational and intervention trials) and umbrella reviews (pooled meta-analyses) confirm that sticking to a healthy diet, especially the MedDiet, can reduce your chances of experiencing depression.

One of the most recent was conducted on behalf of the MooDFOOD consortium, which includes five cohort studies. It found that sticking to a healthy diet was linked to fewer depressive symptoms, although it's still difficult to determine whether poor diet causes depression or vice versa.

The SMILES trial

The cheerily named SMILES (Supporting the Modification of lifestyle in Lowered Emotional States trial), was started in 2012 by Felice Jacka an Australian psychiatrist and head of the Food and Mood Centre at Deakin University. Jacka and her team asked the very simple question, "Can the MedDiet treat depression?"

SMILES recruited people with depression and then randomly assigned them a Befriending or control Group and the Diet Group.

>> **The Befriending control group** met with a member of the research team and chatted about topics they enjoyed, but not related to their mental health.

>> **The Diet group** worked with the dietitian to learn how to follow a modified MedDiet. For example, they ate more fish each week or switched from

chocolate ice cream to natural yogurt with walnuts and honey. They learned that evidence shows that eating in a healthy way, such as the MedDiet, is good for your brain and mental health.

Jacka's study, published in BMC Medicine, found that after three months, one third of people in the diet group achieved remission from major depression, compared to only 8 percent in the social support group, with results linked to dietary changes rather than weight or exercise.

TIP

For depressed people, the biggest help came from changing what they ate.

Connecting diet and dementia

When it comes to protecting yourself from dementia, rather like depression, the evidence is clear: A healthy diet is key!

Clear evidence diet reduces risk for dementia

Go ahead and Google "How do I prevent dementia?," and you find that every reputable global organization or government guideline includes statements along the lines of "Eat a healthy diet."

Even if you're not likely to argue with this fact, consider some of the strongest evidence so far: A 2018 mega impressive umbrella review of meta-analyses, including data from over 12.8 million people! The analysis found that a healthy diet is indeed beneficial for overall mortality and reducing your risk of dementia, heart disease, and diabetes.

Sticking to the MedDiet helps people who are diagnosed with mild cognition impairment (MCI) from progressing further. And those at high risk for developing AD show less AD-like pathology in their brains after they die.

Just as with the relationship between diet and depression, the data indicates potential protective effect. However, distinguishing the direction of causality is complex. Does an unhealthy diet contribute to cognitive decline, or do early cognitive changes affect dietary habits? Or is it a bit of both? And how does AD and people with high genetic risk fit into the picture? And, as I discuss in later chapters, some of the most promising results come from a combination of MedDiet, exercise, stress-management, and social support. One successful trial that combines these is the Finnish Geriatric Intervention Study (FINGER) study (I point that out for you later).

DASH and MIND diets for neuroprotection

A couple of variations of the MedDiet have been put to the test, also with great results for slowing MCI.

>> **The DASH (Dietary Approaches to Stop Hypertension) diet** focuses on reducing sodium (salt) intake and emphasizes fruits, vegetables, whole grains, and lean proteins.

>> **The MIND diet** is a combination of the MedDiet and the DASH diet. And with the added extras of dark leafy greens, such as spinach, and berries, nuts, and fish.

Both diets show promise in protecting against cognitive decline and promoting overall brain health.

Keeping up with the ketogenic diet

The ketogenic diet (KD) is a way of eating that flips the switch on your cell's energy source from using glucose to using ketones. Remember that neurons rely on glucose for their energy. However, when your carb intake is drastically reduced, your liver converts fats into ketone bodies. These cross the blood-brain barrier and serve as an alternative energy source for neurons.

REMEMBER

Ketosis is a state in which the body is using ketone bodies by switching the body's primary metabolism to a fat-based energy source rather than utilizing glucose.

WARNING

Because ketone bodies have anticonvulsant properties, many doctors use the KD as a treatment option for drug-resistant epilepsy, especially in children. However, it's important to note that the KD is not suitable for everyone and should only ever be undertaken with careful medical supervision.

What does the KD diet consist of?

Because the very low carbohydrate KD diet is restrictive, it's hard to stick to and many people don't enjoy the food choices on offer. For people using it to treat health conditions, they may find it hard to comply with, so it's usually considered a last-resort treatment and needs lots of support.

Here's what someone on a keto diet would eat in a day:

>> **Breakfast:** Scrambled eggs with spinach and feta, avocado slices, black coffee or tea (without sugar!)

>> **Lunch:** Grilled chicken, salad with mixed greens, olives, and a high-fat dressing (for example, olive oil and vinegar)

>> **Snack:** A few nuts (for example, almonds or walnuts) and slices of cheese

>> **Dinner:** Baked salmon and steamed broccoli or mashed cauliflower

Ketogenic diet and epilepsy

Epilepsy is a debilitating neurological disorder that I briefly discus in Chapter 4. There are plenty of treatment options such as antiepileptic drugs, deep brain stimulation, and surgery, but they don't work for everyone. For around three out of ten people with epilepsy, their condition is resistant to these therapies. For kids, this can mean they're often missing out on school and sport. For adolescents, they're unable to learn to drive, and, for adults, it affects their work, family life, and overall quality of life.

According to Epilepsy Action Australia, some people with epilepsy respond very well to the KD. It helps reduce seizures for two out of three kids. But it's not free of side effects and plenty of people find it gives them tummy issues such as constipation or diarrhea. And because its missing many vitamins and minerals, children also have to take supplements and need to be closely monitored.

TECHNICAL STUFF

The KD helps reduce epilepsy via a few different biological mechanisms. Its thought ketone bodies balance neurotransmitters by increasing inhibitory GABA and decreasing excitatory glutamate. It may also stabilize ion channels in neurons reducing hyperexcitability. Additionally, it enhances mitochondrial function and ATP production, lowers oxidative stress, and reduces brain inflammation.

Ketogenic diet and serious mental illness

Although data first emerged in mice, the KD has gained popularity online in the last couple of years for its potential benefits in managing schizophrenia, bipolar disorder, and major depressive disorder. But to date, there are mostly case studies and small, but promising, clinical trials.

The idea here is that some psychiatric disorders are due to metabolic dysfunction in the brain. By providing ketone bodies as an alternative fuel to glucose, the KD may treat that metabolic dysfunction. The logic being anything that improves metabolic health is probably going to improve brain health, too.

WARNING

But before the KD can be rolled out to more people, results need to be confirmed in large-scale clinical studies. Starting the KD should only be done in a hospital under the close watch of a doctor and a dietitian, because it can have side effects or make the effects of other drugs worse.

Understanding Neuronal Health: Energy, Metabolism, and Mitochondria

Neurons are your most energy-hungry cells. They're constantly sending and receiving electrical signals, synthesizing, packaging, releasing and recycling neurotransmitters, and pruning and tuning synapses — all of which requires energy in the form of glucose.

Energy requires glucose

Glucose is the primary fuel used by neurons. When your body breaks down the carbohydrates you eat into glucose, it is then ferried to your cells through your bloodstream. Glucose transported inside cells is facilitated by insulin. After inside neurons, glucose undergoes a process called cellular respiration. *Cellular respiration* involves a series of metabolic pathways that convert glucose into adenosine triphosphate (ATP) a process that takes place in your mitochondria.

Why mitochondria matter

Open any textbook and you read that mitochondria are "the powerhouses of the cell." That's because they convert glucose into ATP or energy.

When your mitochondria are healthy, your neurons get the energy they need to perform optimally. When your mitochondria are unhealthy, it can lead to a host of health issues. Dysfunctional mitochondria make less ATP and more highly reactive molecules containing oxygen, which have knock-on effects by damaging the cells they're housed in. Mitochondrial dysfunction is a common feature of many metabolic diseases and can lead to significant neuronal damage over time.

Metabolism: The big picture

Now, zoom your microscope lens out a bit and talk about metabolism.

Metabolism can be defined as the sum of reactions that occur throughout your body and that provide the body with energy. This energy enables an organism to move, grow, develop, and reproduce (and in the case of a brain, think!). All organisms metabolize. Plants capture energy from sunlight, carbon dioxide, and water to make glucose and oxygen, providing energy for growth and development. In muscles, cellular respiration converts glucose into ATP, supplying the energy needed for movement and physical activity.

Metabolic diseases are disorders that disrupt normal metabolism and lead directly to poor health. Some common metabolic diseases in humans include:

>> **Diabetes** affects how your body processes glucose. Two main types of diabetes are Type 1 and Type 2.

- In **Type 1 diabetes**, the body's immune system attacks and destroys the insulin-producing cells in the pancreas, leading to little or no insulin production.

- In **Type 2 diabetes**, the body either doesn't produce enough insulin or becomes resistant to insulin, meaning the cells don't respond effectively to it. This also results in elevated blood sugar levels.

>> **Obesity** or excess body fat increases your risk of various health issues.

>> **Metabolic syndrome** is the name given to a cluster of conditions, including high blood pressure, high blood sugar, excess body fat around the waist, and abnormal cholesterol levels.

How metabolic diseases affect neuronal health

Metabolic dysfunction, such as chronic inflammation and insulin resistance, can negatively impact brain health and contribute to mood disorders. Conditions like diabetes, obesity, and metabolic syndrome are linked to dementia, as high blood sugar damages blood vessels and reduces glucose delivery to neurons.

Excess fat causes inflammation, damaging neurons through oxidative stress and insulin resistance, which limits energy supply to brain cells. Over time, these metabolic issues may lead to cognitive decline and neurodegenerative diseases.

Navigating the Gut-Brain Axis: A Two-Way Street

Have you ever felt butterflies in your stomach before a job interview or giving a talk? That's your brain and gut having a conversation. This two-way conversation is known as the gut-brain axis. It has received a lot of attention in the past decade, some of it valid and some, I'm sorry to say, just hype.

The enteric nervous system

Your digestive tract is the only hollow organ in the body that has developed with its own full nervous system, called the enteric nervous system (ENS). It is a subdivision of the autonomic nervous system but functions without any input from the brain and spinal cord. This ENS controlling gut activities and generating rhythmic contractions moving food from your mouth after you swallow through your entire digestive tract to your anus.

Various types of neurons are involved in gut function including neurons controlling peristalsis (movement) and sensory neurons that report on mechanical (like trapped wind!) and chemical conditions. The independent neurons of the ENS manage motor functions and the secretion of gastrointestinal enzymes, using neurotransmitters like acetylcholine, dopamine, and serotonin to communicate.

The enteric nervous system has about 100 million cells, the same as the spinal cord. This nervous system lies entirely within the gut and can function independently of the central and autonomic nervous systems. Bowel removed from any contact with an animal is capable of rhythmical contractions. Note, removal of the bowel does not result in removal of your "second brain." The enteric nervous system doesn't seem capable of thought as we know it, but it communicates back and forth with our big brain — with profound results.

The gut also receives innervation from:

>> **Parasympathetic nervous system:** The effect of parasympathetic stimulation is to increase gut activity. The proximal half of the nervous system is innervated from the cranial parasympathetic nerve fibers via the vagus.

>> **Sympathetic nervous system:** The sympathetic system's stimulation of the enteric nerves inhibits gut activity. It does this in a minor way with the direct effect of its secreted noradrenaline and in a major way by inhibiting action in the enteric plexuses.

>> **Afferent sensory innervation:** Numerous afferent sensory fibers innervate the gut. Some have their cell bodies in the enteric plexus, and some in the spinal cord. As well as sending information concerning irritation and over-distension, they can also pick up the presence of chemical signals in the gut.

Interoception: Your gut's sense

Interoception is all about perceiving the internal state of your body. So, what I'm talking about here is how your brain processes and understands all those physical signals and sensations you experience, such as heart rate, breathing, body temperature, hunger, thirst, and even discomfort or pain.

Interoception begins in the gut

Interoception begins with interoceptive signals, which include biochemical signals such as hormones and pH levels from your gut, mechanical signals such as stretch or pressure (for example trapped wind!), and electromagnetic signals such as vibration or heat. The brain receives signals from your internal organs through either the vagus nerve or sensory neurons that travel through the spinal cord.

Interoception insights in the insula

The insula is a region of cortex located inside your brain's lateral sulcus. It plays a crucial role in perceiving your internal states. These include sensations of pain, temperature, hunger, thirst, or having a full bladder or an aching back.

TIP

I always remember that INsula is responsible for Interoception as it INterprets INformation from INside your body.

It's interesting how our feelings about our bodies can change over time, becoming stronger or weaker as needed. When your interoceptive sense is dysfunctional, it can mean that you're having trouble correctly detecting and understanding your body's internal states. Take irritable bowel syndrome (IBS) as an example. People with IBS have what's called visceral hypersensitivity. This means that they probably pay a lot of attention to their stomach problems, become hypervigilant, and their insula may interpret what's happening in their belly in an unhelpful way.

The gut-brain-microbiome axis

Adding another layer of complexity to the brain-gut conversation, the gut hosts a microbiome. This microbiome comprises trillions of bacteria and other microorganisms.

John Cryan, an Irish neuroscientist working in the field, likened gut-brain communication to Downton Abbey-like upstairs/downstairs communication:

> "The upstairs and the downstairs need each other to survive. From a distance, it looks like they are living completely separate and they don't have much to do with one another. But when things start going wrong downstairs that filters on upstairs. It's the same with the gut and the brain. If there is something wrong with your microbiome, it's going to filter on upstairs in the brain, too."

Most studies of the gut-microbiome are in mice

The first good evidence that gut microbes influence brain chemistry can be traced back to 1986. A study famously (well, famous to some neuroscientists!) observed that germ-free (GF) or gnotobiotic mice had lower baseline levels of the neuromodulator histamine in their hypothalamus compared to conventional "germy" controls.

GF mice are born and raised in conditions that ensure they're living without a gut microbiome. They're delivered via Caesarean section ensuring they're not exposed to their mother's vaginal microbiome and grow up in sterile cages fostered by germ-free foster mothers. Studies on these unusually reared GF mice show the following:

>> The absence of microbial colonization causes abnormalities in neuron maturation at both the brain and gut nervous system.

>> They have altered neurotransmitter expression as well as gastrointestinal sensory/motor abnormalities.

>> Their hypothalamic-pituitary-adrenal (HPA) axis (part of the physiological stress-response system) develops abnormally.

>> Display an increased stress response.

>> Replacing their gut microbiome helps their stress-response system to return to a healthy baseline for mice.

This study demonstrates the extraordinary ability of gut bacteria to influence brain chemistry and behavior. And it offers an intriguing new perspective on how the food you eat may have a significant impact on your mental health. However, (sorry, I must include a caveat!) it is critical to realize that these findings, as cool as they are, are based on research conducted in mice rather than humans.

Gut microbiota, depression, and AD (Alzheimer's Disease)

Take a look at a few of the more fascinating research studies in humans, then come back down to earth to look at what it all means therapeutically or practically for you on a daily basis. Because, despite the excitement, most scientists and physicians remain rightly cautious.

A landmark study in 2014 titled *Correlation between the Human Fecal Microbiota and Depression* highlighted changes in gut microbiota composition in patients with depression. Yes, in the name of science, they tested people's poo! The study noted an overrepresentation of the bacterial sub-family Bacteroidales and a reduction in the family Lachnospiraceae in people with depression compared to healthy people. As you can imagine, this study sparked off enormous interest in the field of psychobiotics.

A 2023 study published in the journal *Brain* made quite the splash with its ick factor. Researchers transplanted the fecal microbiome from people with AD into microbiota-depleted (germ-free) young rats. (Yes, you read that correctly: Poo was transplanted from people to rats). The results showed that rats receiving the AD patient poo transplants showed changes in their behaviors linked to reduced hippocampal neurogenesis. Importantly, the degree of the rat's behavioral changes correlated with the cognitive scores of their human donors. In other words, the worse the cognitive impairment in the AD patients, the more pronounced the impairments in the rats. And yes, while it may sound "ick," this research highlights the significant impact of gut health on brain function.

A role for probiotics in brain health

If the gut-brain link intrigues people, then the gut-brain-microbiome is their newfound obsession. Probiotics, found in fermented foods like yogurt, kefir, and sauerkraut, are popular for gut health, but their role in brain health is still being explored. While it would be amazing if a probiotic pill or kimchi could protect against depression or Alzheimer's, it's not that simple, as defining a "healthy microbiome" is tricky due to individual differences like stress, nutrition, and illness.

Research is ongoing, with projects like American Gut and British Gut working to establish what a healthy microbiome looks like. Though enjoying fermented foods as part of a balanced diet is beneficial, current studies on probiotics for dementia show no significant effects, and findings on depression are mixed. The concept of "psycho-biotics" for mental health shows promise but remains in early stages.

Without this baseline, we're left relying on anecdote rather than carefully gathered data.

Enjoying yogurt, kefir, kimchi, and even sauerkraut as part of a healthy diet won't do you any harm. The field of "psycho-biotics" for depression shows promise, but not promises yet!

A theory of everything?

WARNING

Rather entertainingly, John Cryan and Tim Dinan, the two prominent neuroscientists in this field, have commented that just as physicists have been searching for a comprehensive "theory of everything," the gut has become "a theory of everything" in medicine.

A lot of so-called lifestyle diseases have some common underlying factors such as immune dysregulation, a wonky stress response, and lifestyle choices such as diet, exercise, and alcohol or smoking. Research on the gut-brain connection is still in its infancy, and to date, no magical edible gut tonics, yogurt drinks have shown any promise as a cure for AD. But watch this space!

Answering Common Brain Health-Nutrition Questions

To conclude this chapter, I'll do my best to answer common questions involving nutrition and brain health that I'm asked.

Is coffee good for your brain?

I have good news for coffee lovers: higher coffee intake (around three cups of coffee a day) is linked to a reduced risk of AD, PD, multiple sclerosis (MS), some cancers, and slows mild cognitive decline. And it's not just your brain that benefits from coffee. Research from the New England Journal of Medicine also shows that coffee drinkers are less likely to die from heart disease, respiratory disease, stroke, injuries, diabetes, and infections, although it doesn't protect against cancer.

Caffeine works by blocking adenosine receptors in the brain, which helps improve mood and alertness. Additionally, coffee is rich in antioxidants, which offer protective benefits. Just remember, moderation is key, especially later in the day to avoid sleep disruption.

So yes, coffee is neuroprotective, but don't overdo it!

Is red wine really good for you?

Red wine has had its fair share of praise and criticism. Some meta-analyses show that moderate red wine consumption (usually as part of the MedDiet) can reduce the risk of dementia thanks to polyphenols such as resveratrol, which have anti-oxidant and anti-inflammatory properties.

However, even moderate drinking can lead to cognitive decline, brain atrophy, and increased dementia risk. The most recent data from the U.K. BioBank find even one standard drink or two a day is linked to smaller overall brain volume. One or two drinks also seriously disrupts healthy sleep architecture (the cycles of sleep you follow over the course of a night).

REMEMBER

So a little red wine shared with friends may be fun on occasion, but too much is definitely toxic to brain health.

Can intermittent fasting benefit brain health?

Intermittent fasting (IF) is generating buzz for its potential brain health benefits, involving cycles of fasting and eating, like the 16:8 method where you fast for 16 hours and eat within an 8-hour window. This can naturally reduce calorie intake, contributing to improved metabolic health and potentially supporting brain function.

Animal studies suggest IF may extend lifespan and promote good health, with early human research indicating it could reduce depression symptoms and Alzheimer's risk by boosting brain-derived neurotrophic factor (BDNF) and reducing inflammation. It also encourages autophagy, where cells clean out damaged components to regenerate. However, IF isn't a one-size-fits-all solution, and it's not recommended for everyone.

Does fish oil help with childhood learning?

Omega-3 fatty acids are essential for brain function, especially during fetal and early childhood development. Traditional diets high in fish (like the Japanese and Norwegian diets) are often associated with lower rates of neurodegenerative diseases and improved cognition.

The idea that fish oil supplements can boost children's cognitive abilities or academic performance is appealing but unproven. While some small studies showed improvements in reading and behavior, larger studies failed to replicate these findings. Omega-3s might help some kids with specific learning challenges, but fish oil pills certainly won't teach children to read!

Is sugar as addictive as cocaine?

The claim that sugar is as addictive as cocaine is compelling yet controversial.

Both sugar and cocaine increase dopamine levels, creating pleasure and cravings, but sugar cravings typically don't have the life-altering impact of drug addiction. As the late British health journalist Michael Mosley humorously pointed out, sugar addicts don't usually eat spoonfuls of plain sugar.

In lab rats, sugar can cause cravings similar to those for cocaine, especially in certain settings. However, calling sugar an "addiction" has been critiqued for downplaying the severity of true addiction, which leads to serious life impairments, unlike most people's sugar cravings.

Chapter **13**

Moving Your Body for Brain Health

M odern science and ancient wisdom agree: How you eat, move, sleep, form relationships, and find meaning shapes your brain's growth, thinking, feelings, and aging. And guess what? Physical exercise tops the list of brain-boosting activities.

In this chapter, you'll discover how your brain evolved "on foot" (not on the couch). And you'll find out exactly how exercise gives your brain a pep talk, getting it pumped and ready for whatever life throws at it. Whether it's a brisk walk, tough gym session, dance party with your friends, or even pottering around the garden, you'll learn how movement powers up your brain health and mental well-being.

Getting Brain Gains from Physical Activity

Strong evidence shows regular physical activity improves brain function, lowers mental health issues, and cuts the risk of cognitive decline and dementia. Dig into why this is true through the lens of evolution.

Your brain evolved on the move

Around two million years ago, our ancestors shifted from a chill, sedentary life to a dynamic hunting and gathering one. This lifestyle demanded a lot of walking, lifting, stretching, and climbing. Our bodies and brains evolved to thrive with this activity level. So, it's no wonder we need exercise to stay sharp.

Movement is more than just physical

Some scientists suggest our brains evolved not just to think and feel but to control movement. This concept means we process information and emotions better when we're active.

Cognitive neuroscientist David Raichlen proposes that human evolutionary history as "cognitively engaged endurance athletes" ties our brain health to movement. When you become sedentary, your brain "downsizes" functionally to save energy, leading to age-related brain shrinkage. He argues the converse is also true: Human cognition thrives when you're goal-oriented, a little bit hungry, and on the move. When we're active, we plan, recall, navigate, focus, and cooperate, keeping our brain sharp and energized. So to stay at your cognitive best, embrace your roots and keep moving!

Sedentary living and brain health

In today's world, you may find yourself unwittingly leading a sedentary lifestyle. You may spend long hours sitting at your desk, driving your car, or relaxing in front of a screen (or, like me, six months writing a *For Dummies* book!). This less-than-ideal shift away from regular daily movement has significant implications not only for your physical health but also for your brain health. And this goes for every age and every life stage.

According to the Australian Department of Health guidelines, sedentary behavior refers to periods of inactivity where you are sitting or lying down, excluding sleep. This includes time spent inactive at school, work, during travel, or while relaxing. Physical activity is any movement that gets your body moving, makes you breathe faster, and increases your heart rate.

Many forms of sedentary behavior involve screens, such as:

>> Working or doing homework on a computer

>> Playing video games

>> Scrolling through social media

>> Watching movies

But there are various types of physical activity, including:

>> **Incidental activity:** Activities such as mowing the lawn, cleaning the house, or walking to the bus stop

>> **Exercise:** Planned or structured physical activities, such as going to the gym, swimming, or jogging each day

>> **Sport:** Engaging in sports such as rugby, netball, or tennis

>> **Muscle strengthening activities:** Exercises such as weight training or bodyweight exercises

Physical activity can be performed at different intensities, including:

>> **Light:** Activities that you may do without much thought, such as strolling in the garden, getting dressed, or stretching

>> **Moderate:** Activities that require some effort but aren't too strenuous, such as bike riding or brisk walking

>> **Vigorous:** Activities that make you out of breath and sweat, such as jogging, jumping jacks, or doing sit-ups

Both sedentary behavior *and* lack of physical inactivity can increase the risk of health issues such as diabetes, heart disease, depression, and dementia.

Government guidelines

Many governments and health organizations provide clear guidelines on physical activity. For example, the WHO recommends that adults engage in at least 150 minutes of moderate-intensity aerobic physical activity or 75 minutes of vigorous-intensity activity per week, combined with muscle-strengthening activities on two or more days a week. Moderate-intensity is doing any activity that gets your heart rate up and makes you breathe faster, but you can still talk while doing it — such as walking up a gentle hill, dancing, or riding your bike.

Because I live in Australia, I looked up the Australian Government Department of Health guidelines on physical activity. Here is a summary for people of different ages:

For children and adolescents

Because kid's physical activity levels have decreased, sedentary behaviors have increased, and sleep deprivation has become common, the 2019 updated Australian government recommendations advocate for a 24-hour integrated movement.

TIP

Guidelines recommend at least 60 minutes of moderate to vigorous daily activity for those aged 5–17, mixing aerobic exercises with muscle and bone-strengthening activities. Screen time should be limited to 2 hours per day, and children should aim for 9-11 hours of sleep (5-13 years) or 8-10 hours (14–17 years), with consistent wake-up times.

For young and middle-aged adults

When developing the activity guidelines for Australians aged 18 to 64, the 2012 review of evidence determined that any physical activity is better than doing none.

TIP

Guidelines recommend you start with any physical activity if you're inactive and aim for 150-300 minutes of moderate aerobic exercise weekly, alongside strength training twice a week. Break up long sitting periods with light activity.

For older adults

Given their high risk of mortality and various health issues, sedentary older adults stand to benefit the most from increasing and maintaining physical activity.

TIP

Here's my take on the recommendations:

>> Stay active with any form of physical movement, no matter your age or health.

>> Incorporate various exercises daily, including strength, balance, and flexibility.

>> Aim for at least 30 minutes of exercise most days.

>> Start slow and increase activity gradually if you're new or returning to exercise.

>> Continue vigorous physical activity suited to your capability.

>> Break up long periods of sitting as often as possible.

Analyzing Evidence for Exercise for Brain Health

Walk through some more recent and interesting evidence that may help convince you of the brain health benefits of adopting the previous Aussie guidelines.

Playing their way to childhood brain health

When it comes to children and screens, the impact on brain health is unsurprising! Preschool kids need energetic play to develop self-regulation, which is crucial for both their mental health and academic success. Like all young mammals, they naturally do this through play.

WARNING

However, as children grow older, they often become less active and fall into sedentary habits, often due to increased screen time. This issue, known as *technoference*, suggests that balancing screen time with physical activity is key for cognitive development and better academic performance.

Being a couch potato can harm the healthy development of executive functioning skills. (For a review of the development of executive functioning in childhood, check out Chapter 6). While computer gaming, especially when played with friends, can enhance certain executive skills, excessive passive TV watching is linked to attention problems in school.

Looking at the classroom evidence

By now, you know I love diving into epic meta-analyses because they provide me with a solid foundation for making brain health recommendations!

TECHNICAL STUFF

A 2023 meta-analysis published in the *Educational Psychology Review* examined 92 randomized control trials involving over 25,000 children aged five to 12 to investigate the effects of physical activity on their cognition and academic performance. Physical activity was broadly defined and included everything from doing jumping jacks while counting in math class to playing soccer at recess. Physical activity significantly improved children's on-task behavior and had small but positive effects on working memory, fluid intelligence, and creativity, particularly when incorporating activities like dance. However, no notable improvements were observed in attention, inhibitory control, or overall academic outcome.

TIP

In essence, getting kids moving not only keeps them physically fit but also gives their brains a boost, especially when the activities are fun!

Treating mood disorders with exercise

The evidence is clear: Exercise is a game-changer for mental health prevention and treatment.

Current clinical practice guidelines now recommend exercise as a frontline mental health intervention. Take a quick look at some of the latest reviews.

TECHNICAL STUFF

In 2023, a massive umbrella review analyzed 97 systematic reviews, covering over 1,000 trials and 128,000 participants! This comprehensive research included healthy adults, people with mental health issues such as anxiety and depression, and those with chronic diseases. The findings were striking: Exercise significantly improved symptoms of mild-to-moderate depression, anxiety, and psychological distress, often more effectively than standard care such as talk therapy or medications.

Some differences in the types of exercise that helped different mood disorders are:

>> **Depression:** Resistance exercise (such as lifting weights) had the most significant impact on reducing depression.

>> **Anxiety:** Yoga and other mind-body exercises had the most significant impact on reducing anxiety.

Calculating the sweet spot: Exercise type, timing, and frequency

TECHNICAL STUFF

In (yes, yet another!) mega-impressive study, researchers examined the relationship between exercise and mental health burden by analyzing data from over 1.2 million Americans. Because all those people did a lot of different types of exercise, everything from walking and gardening to cycling, team sports, snow and water sports. This meant the researchers could zoom in on this relationship between good mental health and exercise and they asked questions such as:

>> What type of physical activity or exercised did you spend the most time doing during the past month?

>> How long do you exercise for? And how often?

>> Now thinking about your mental health, which includes stress, depression, and problems with emotions, for how many days during the past 30 days was your mental health not good?

As the lead author of the study Adam Chekrod tweeted, "The punchline was clear. . . people who exercised had about 40 percent better mental health than people who didn't exercise. . ."

Here's a summary of their key findings:

>> Exercise improves mental health by 40 percent compared to not exercising.

>> Team sports offer the biggest mental health benefits due to social interaction.

>> Even walking or housework is beneficial.

>> Optimal session duration is 45 minutes for best results.

>> Exercising 3–5 times a week is ideal for mental health.

>> Over-exercising (more than 6 times weekly or sessions longer than 90 minutes) can harm mental health.

Motiving people with depression

Feeling motivated to exercise when you're dealing with depression is tough. The two go hand in hand. Because even small steps can make a big difference, it is useful to consider what you are able to do.

TIP

Here are some ideas to get you moving:

>> Start with manageable goals, such as a 10-minute walk or some simple stretches. Gradually, increase the time and intensity.

>> Consider exercising with a friend or joining a group class for social support and accountability.

>> Look for structured exercise programs designed for people with depression; these can provide routine and extra encouragement.

REMEMBER

Reintroducing enjoyable activities, including exercise, can help lift your mood over time.

Battling cognitive decline and dementia with exercise

In the never-ending healthcare quest to fend off dementia, plenty of studies have spotlighted the impressive role of physical activity and avoiding a sedentary life-style. In Chapter 8, I discuss the Lancet Commission on Dementia Prevention and

Intervention that identifies physical inactivity as one of the 14 modifiable risk factors for dementia. You can gently meander through some of that data here.

Preventing mild cognitive impairment (MCI) and dementia

An extensive 2023 umbrella review of various meta-analyses reveal just how crucial exercise is. The findings are summed up as follows:

>> Regular exercise significantly reduces the risk of developing Alzheimer's Disease, with 150 minutes of moderate activity per week recommended by the WHO.

>> For MCI, exercise, especially strength training and aerobic workouts, improves cognitive function and overall quality of life.

Heart pumping or leg lifting?

With so many ways to stay fit and active, it's natural to wonder which type of exercise may be the most beneficial. According to a 2023 meta-analysis, resistance exercise and multi-component exercise stand out as particularly effective for managing mild cognitive impairment (MCI).

>> Resistance exercise, which focuses on building strength, is particularly effective at slowing cognitive decline, especially in dementia patients.

>> Multi-component exercise, combining aerobic, resistance, and balance training, is most effective for preventing declines in cognition and executive function in people with MCI.

WARNING

If you or a loved one is not able to exercise or at risk of falls, talk to your doctor about getting help from an exercise physiologist. They can recommend tailored exercise routines that are supervised and integrated into daily activities to help stay healthy.

Decoding the Exercise Effect

You may well ask, why does exercise pack such a punch for brain health? Here is a summary of the many varied biological mechanisms pathways via which physical activity gets into your neurons and synapses to improve brain health:

- >> **Heart health:** Exercise enhances blood flow and oxygen delivery to the brain, nourishes brain cells, supports waste removal, and reduces the risk of cognitive decline and neurodegenerative diseases.

- >> **Blood vessel health:** Exercise stimulates the formation of new blood vessels in the brain, ensures a steady supply of oxygen and nutrients to brain tissues, and improves brain plasticity for learning and memory.

- >> **Metabolic health/Diabetes risk:** Exercise improves insulin sensitivity, regulates blood sugar levels, reduces the risk of type 2 diabetes, and supports proper glucose metabolism essential for brain energy.

- >> **Inflammation:** Exercise reduces levels of pro-inflammatory cytokines, promotes the production of anti-inflammatory molecules, and supports brain health while protecting against cognitive decline.

- >> **Stress response:** Exercise lowers levels of cortisol (the stress hormone), enhances mood through endorphin release, improves cognitive function, and fosters resilience.

- >> **Neurogenesis in hippocampus:** Exercise stimulates the creation of new neurons in the hippocampus (in mice and rats; the jury is out on humans).

- >> **Brain-derived neurotrophic factor (BDNF):** Exercise promotes the growth and differentiation of new neurons and synapses, boosts neuroplasticity for memory and learning, and is associated with improved overall cognitive function.

- >> **Myokine release:** Muscles release messaging molecules known as myokines during exercise (including the newly discovered, irisin). Irisin acts via BDNF to promote neurogenesis and protect against neurodegeneration, highlighting muscle-brain communication benefits.

- >> **Endorphin release:** The so-called "runner's high" is real! Endorphins released during exercise act as natural painkillers, reduce stress and anxiety, and the mood boost makes you want to go back for more.

- >> **Social-cognitive resilience:** Exercise often involves social interaction, improving social skills, reducing feelings of loneliness, and providing mental stimulation to enhance brain health.

- >> **Improved mood:** Leads to healthier choices, which reduces symptoms of depression and anxiety, leads to healthier lifestyle choices (better nutrition, consistent sleep), and creates a positive feedback loop for mental well-being.

SKELETAL MUSCLE AND MYOKINES

Scientists now understand that skeletal muscle is an endocrine organ, producing and releasing molecules that act locally or throughout the body, much like hormones. Myokines are a type of signaling molecule made and released by skeletal muscle cells during exercise. One such myokine, Irisin — named after Iris, the Greek goddess and messenger of the gods — may prove to be a crucial link between muscle tissue and other organs, such as the brain. While our understanding of Irisin's functions is still developing, it is known to help regulate neurogenesis through its interaction with BDNF.

Implementing Movement into Your Everyday Life

Both you and I will inevitably have those days when the couch looks more inviting than a walk or a workout. On those days, remember that any movement is better than none (even I've been known to get up from the couch, squat three times and consider my daily workout done!).

From a neurobiological standpoint, habits are the most powerful tools you have for behavior change. Unlike motivation, which can be fleeting or hard to muster up, habits embed behaviors into your daily routine.

REMEMBER

To incorporate exercise into your daily life, start small and build gradually. Begin with manageable activities such as a 10-minute walk after lunch or a quick set of push-ups before your evening shower. As these activities become habitual, you can increase the intensity or duration. The key is consistency and making the exercise feel like a natural part of your day.

Over time, these small changes add up, and you find that exercise is no longer a chore but a regular, enjoyable part of your routine.

As I discuss in the following sections, by understanding and applying the habit loop, incorporating "If-Then" planning, using habit stacking, creating environmental nudges, and leveraging social support networks, you can turn daily leg strength training into a natural and automatic part of your routine. Happy exercising!

Harnessing the power of habits

REMEMBER

As a human, you're a creature of habit. You may not realize it, but from the time you wake up in the morning and until you fall asleep in the evening, you're acting and thinking according to automated learned behaviors known as habits. Many of your actions and thoughts today were the same as they were yesterday and will be repeated again tomorrow.

Changing behavior through habits

Habits form when a behavior you repeat often enough shifts from being a deliberate action that requires motivation and concentration into an automatic response you do without much effort. Once formed, they make you efficient, as they enable you to perform tasks with minimal conscious effort.

WARNING

However, their inflexibility can make adapting to new situations or learning new skills challenging. Often, bad habits are the root cause of your failed attempts at behavior change.

Researchers have noted that nearly half — around 43 percent — of your actions and thoughts are habitual, repeated daily in the same time or place. Now, imagine how beneficial it would be to have daily movement as one of your habits! By incorporating regular physical activity into your routine, you can improve your efficiency and well-being without much extra effort. This habit of daily movement can significantly enhance your overall health and cognitive function.

TECHNICAL STUFF

The brain likes to be as efficient as possible, so it actively reduces the cognitive load required to perform the behavior, turned it into a habit, and making it easier to maintain over time. This process involves the basal ganglia, a part of the brain responsible for habit formation, which allows actions to occur with minimal conscious thought. Essentially, habits free up your cognitive resources.

Understanding the habit loop

Creating a habit of daily exercise can be a game-changer for your health. The habit loop consists of four key components: cue, craving, response, and reward. Here's a breakdown of how you can turn an activity, such as leg strength training, into a daily habit by using the concept of a habit loop.

>> **Cue:** This trigger or context initiates your habit. It can be an external stimulus (such as the sight of your workout shoes) or an internal one (such as feeling restless after sitting for too long). One idea is to put your workout mat and dumbbells where you can easily see them, perhaps near your bed or in the living room. This visual cue will remind you to exercise.

>> **Craving:** This concept is the desire or motivation to perform the behavior. For example, you may crave the feeling of accomplishment or the endorphin rush after exercising. Try to focus on the brain health benefits you gain, not just stronger legs, and more energy, but the BDNF that is trigged by muscles moving! Visualizing these benefits can increase your motivation.

>> **Response:** This component is the actual behavior you perform. In your case, it can be performing leg strength exercises. Start with simple routines such as squats or lunges. Set a specific time each day, like right after you wake up or during your lunch break, to make it easier to remember.

>> **Reward:** This component is the positive outcome you get from the behavior. It can be a sense of relief, improved mood, or better health over time. After your workout, treat yourself to something enjoyable. It can be a delicious smoothie, a few minutes of relaxation, or watching an episode of your favorite Netflix show. Over time, the intrinsic reward of feeling stronger and more energized will also kick in.

TIP

By consistently applying the habit loop components — Cue, Craving, Response, and Reward — you can seamlessly integrate leg strength training into your daily routine, transforming it into a lasting and beneficial habit.

Using "If-Then" planning

Contrary to the popular belief that habits take 21 days to form (wouldn't that solve everything!), research on habit formation among university students found it often takes around 66 days and can take up to 256 days (about eight months), for a new behavior to become habitual.

This means it's normal and natural to sometimes feel discouraged if your learned behaviors don't become habits straight away. One mind trick you can use is "If-Then" planning. It's a way to manage your excuses or barriers to exercise in advance! Here's how you can incorporate "If-Then" planning into your leg strength for brain health protocol:

TIP

Create a simple plan that outlines a clear trigger and a specific action. For example:

>> *"IF* it's 6:30PM and I'm watching the evening news, *THEN* I'll do ten minutes of leg strength exercises."

>> *"IF* I start brewing a morning coffee, *THEN* I'll do ten squats and five lunges each leg."

By creating these "If-Then" plans, you make it easier to follow through with your exercise routine because you've already made the decision to do so and the plan is in place.

Stacking habits

Habit stacking is another technique to use that involves linking or stacking your new habit on top of existing one. Here's how you can use habit stacking in the context of your leg-strengthening routine.

TIP

If you already have a morning coffee routine (and let's face it, caffeine dependency can be very helpful here!), you can stack your new habit onto your coffee habit or another daily activity. For example:

>> "While I brew my morning coffee, I'll also do ten squats."

>> "While I'm brushing my teeth, I'll balance on one leg."

By stacking your leg strength exercises onto a habit you already do daily without needing to be motivated to do so, you create a seamless and automatic transition into your new routine.

Environmental nudging

Environmental nudges are changes you make to your surroundings (such as your home or office) to encourage desired behaviors and discourage undesired ones. The classic public health example of an environmental nudge is Australia's success in nudging its citizens to stop smoking by mandating all cigarettes be sold in plain packages and hidden from view in shops.

TIP

Here's how you can use environmental nudges to support your exercise habit.

>> **Place your workout gear (mat, dumbbells, resistance bands) in a visible and easily accessible spot.** Don't hide them away as if they're a pack of Australian cigarettes!

>> **Rearrange your living space** to create a designated workout area.

>> **Keep your workout clothes in a convenient location,** such as next to your bed or in the bathroom, to make it easier to change into them. Or, if you're really keen for early morning exercise, sleep in them!

>> **Get a dog.** Studies show that dog owners walk about 200 minutes more per week than those without dogs. A wet nose nudge, soulful eyes, and the joy of watching your furry friend race around the dog park make staying active so much easier.

These small adjustments in your environment can significantly increase the likelihood of you sticking to your exercise routine.

Incorporating social support networks

Friends: They'll be there for you. Social support networks involve leveraging the encouragement and accountability provided by other people. For example, if you tell a friend you'll meet them at the beach for a swim, or at the dog park for a walk, you're more likely to go through with that plan because you don't want to let them down.

TIP

Here's how you can get by with a little help from you friends:

>> Find a workout buddy who can join you in your leg strength exercises, walks, swims, or gym sessions.

>> Join a fitness class where you can share your progress and challenges.

>> Shout it out to all your friends and family! Tell them about your exercise goals so they can offer support and encouragement.

Having a supportive network can provide motivation, accountability, and a sense of camaraderie, making it easier to maintain your exercise habits.

MY MOVEMENT THROUGHOUT THE WEEK

I'm lucky enough to live on the Northern Beaches of Sydney, Australia. In the last chapter, I encouraged you to take an imaginary trip to Italy. Now, I'd like you to accompany me as I move through my week. Moving is especially important because I'm spending plenty of time being sedentary writing *Brain Health For Dummies!* One way I counteract all the sitting is to set a 30-minute rolling alarm on my phone. This reminds to stand up and move about.

Now, imagine us starting the week with a 7 a.m. ocean swim at Manly Beach with the locals who are welcoming and supportive to newcomers. We can marvel at the cool sea life and admire the surfers paddling out into the early morning sun. Later in the week, we can head to the gym, where I either lift heavy weights or stretch out in a Pilates class. Sometimes we jog — or let's be honest, shuffle — along the beach. On another day, we can march on the treadmill together, laughing at reality TV shows. Most evenings, we take my dog for a walk (well, he'll sprint) through the local bushland. By the weekend, we are dancing (awkwardly, in my case) at the back of a community theatre dance ensemble with other midlife moms.

As you move alongside me, you discover I don't take *myself* too seriously, but I take the enjoyment of different forms of exercise for brain health very seriously! Your brain will seriously thank you, too.

Chapter **14**

Sleeping Your Way to Better Brain Health

You (ideally!) spend a significant amount of each day sleeping. In this chapter, you start to unravel the mysteries of why you sleep and its profound significance for brain health.

In your quest for better brain health, sleep is not just a luxury but a necessity. Just as a doctor prescribes medication if you're sick, consider sleep as your nightly prescription for optimal brain function. Ensuring you get quality sleep every night is one of the most effective strategies you can adopt for maintaining cognitive performance, emotional stability, and overall well-being.

REMEMBER

A good night's sleep is the foundation upon which all other aspects of health are built. In this chapter, I equip you with a toolkit for better sleep and better brain health.

Understanding Sleep's Significance for Brain Health

Humans spend a third of their lives sleeping — 30 years in total if you reach 90. This fact underscores sleep's significance. Without sleep, your brain health and well-being rapidly deteriorate.

Asking the big question: Why do we need to sleep?

REMEMBER

Sleep is essential for growth, development, rest, repair, and maintaining healthy neural function. Think about the last time you skipped a night or two of sleep — you probably felt irritable, emotionally sensitive, had difficulty concentrating, made mistakes, needed coffee, and felt an overwhelming urge to catch up on sleep. Chronic lack of sleep over weeks, months, or years is linked to serious health problems such as anxiety, depression, heart disease, diabetes, and dementia.

Several plausible theories have been proposed to explain why you need to sleep. No one or two of these theories thoroughly explain why you sleep; they probably all contribute.

>> **The Inactivity Theory** proposes that staying inactive at night keeps you hidden and safe from predators.

>> **The Energy Conservation Theory** suggests that you sleep to decrease energy expenditure.

>> **The Restorative Theory** posits that sleep allows cellular repair and rejuvenation.

>> **The Glymphatic Cleaning Theory** suggests that the brain's glial-regulated lymphatic (glymphatic) system, activated during sleep, purges the day's metabolic waste. However, a 2024 study called this theory into question, finding that the glymphatic system is more active during wake than sleep.

>> **The Memory Processing Theory** is based on the fact that sleep processes and organizes memories, ensuring they are accessible for future recall.

REMEMBER

Instead of asking why you need to sleep, perhaps you should consider if any aspect of your health and well-being doesn't benefit from a good night's sleep!

Deciphering the sleep cycle

Just as different types of food make up a well-balanced, healthy meal, different types or stages of sleep are necessary for a healthy night's slumber.

Studying sleep with polysomnography

Sleep scientists and doctors track and record sleep using *polysomnography*. This technique records data on brain activity using EEG, eye and muscle activity using movement sensors, and other metrics such as blood oxygen levels, heart rate, and breathing (see Figure 14-1). Polysomnography is particularly useful in clinical sleep studies where diagnosing sleep disorders is necessary.

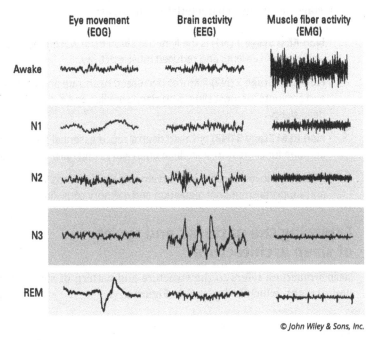

© John Wiley & Sons, Inc.

FIGURE 14-1: Stages of sleep recorded by polysomnography.

Based on polysomnography data, scientists now talk about four stages of sleep: Rapid Eye Movement (REM) sleep and three stages of non–Rapid Eye Movement (NREM) sleep. Every 90 minutes or so during the night, you cycle through the various stages of sleep, from lighter NREM to deeper NREM and back again to REM.

REM, NREM, AND EEG

EEG recordings capture the synchronized activity of millions of pyramidal neurons in the brain's cortex as they periodically depolarize and hyperpolarize during sleep. Like a microphone picking up a crowd's roar at a football game, EEG measures the collective electrical activity, not individual neurons. This synchronized firing, modulated by deeper brain structures like the thalamus and hippocampus, creates the characteristic brain wave patterns of NREM slow waves and REM rapid rhythms.

Stages of sleep

Each stage has unique characteristics and roles:

1. **Non-REM Stage 1 (N1)** is the light transition from wakefulness to sleep with slow eye movements and reduced muscle activity.

2. **Non-REM Stage 2 (N2)** features decreased heart rate and body temperature, and accounts for most sleep with sleep spindles and K-complexes signaling deep sleep.

3. **Non-REM Stage 3 (N3)** or called deep sleep, is essential for recovery and immune function, with slow delta brain waves and hard-to-wake conditions.

4. **REM sleep** involves rapid eye movements, vivid dreams, muscle paralysis, and supports emotional regulation and memory consolidation.

Exploring the patterns and cycles of sleep architecture

Sleep architecture refers to the structure and pattern of sleep cycles throughout a typical night, which is depicted in Figure 14-2.

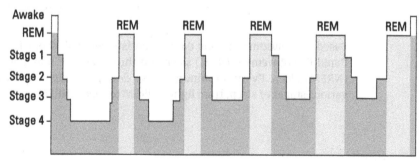

FIGURE 14-2:
Sleep architecture.

© John Wiley & Sons, Inc.

Sleep architecture includes the sequence and duration of the sleep stages — NREM stages 1, 2, and 3, followed by REM sleep — and how they repeat cyclically throughout the night. Each cycle lasts about 90 to 120 minutes, with a typical night involving multiple cycles. The cycles are shorter in babies and young children: Around 60 minutes.

As you can see in Figure 14-3. sleep patterns and needs vary significantly throughout different stages of life. Understanding these variations helps explain how sleep supports overall health and development.

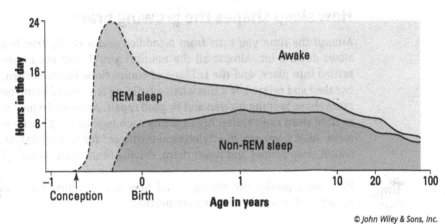

© John Wiley & Sons, Inc.

FIGURE 14-3: Sleep architecture change during the lifespan.

Messing up your sleep architecture

Disruptions in your sleep architecture can significantly affect mental and physical health. Here are some factors that may interfere with healthy sleep patterns:

>> Alcohol, coffee, tea, certain medications, and large evening meals

>> Stress, anxiety, sleep disorders

>> Bedroom environment including electronic devices emitting blue light, temperature extremes

>> Lack of exercise

>> Aging

Understanding and mitigating these factors can help you maintain a healthy sleep architecture, ensuring you get restorative and uninterrupted sleep each night.

Sleep: The price you pay for brain plasticity

Imagine your developing brain is a garden and sleep is the gardener. When the garden is newly established, the gardener's job is to nurture the young plants, helping them to grow strong and flourish. As the garden matures, the gardener switches to carefully pruning the plants, cutting back the overgrowth so that the healthiest, most useful plants have room to thrive. Like a well-tended garden, your brain uses sleep to help it flourish and grow and later sculpt and refine, ensuring it stays healthy and functions at its best.

How sleep shapes the growing brain

Around the time you turn from a toddler into a child, your brain development slows down a bit. Almost all the neurons you'll ever need have been born and settled into place, and the trillions of connections between them are ready to be tweaked and refined. It's like when a building is finished being built, and now it's more about keeping it clean and in good repair. Around age four or five, the NREM to REM sleep ratio shifts, highlighting each type of sleep's role in brain development. REM sleep acts like "electrical fertilizer" for new neural connections, while NREM sleep prunes and tunes them, driving brain maturation.

REM sleep guides the wiring up of new neural connections, and NREM sleep prunes and tunes the existing connections.

Simply put, growing brains need sleep. Babies, toddlers, and even teenagers need lots of sleep to develop, learn, and stay healthy, just like plants require water.

Sleep's role in learning and memory

Brain development is not the only thing that needs sleep. Sleep is the mechanism by which the lessons we absorb during the day are transformed into memories. Sleep is responsible for *memory consolidation* — the process of turning a temporary, unstable memory into one that does not fade over time.

Sleep also helps you learn new skills. When you learn something new, such as riding a bike or your times tables, your brain is busy creating new connections between neurons. At first, riding a bike feels awkward because the neuronal connections are new and not well-worn, but with practice, it becomes second nature.

In a series of clever experiments, Harvard University psychiatrist and sleep scientist Robert Stickgold showed sleep within 30 hours of learning a new skill is absolutely required for learning new skills. In some of his experiments, he used sleep deprivation to prove his point.

TIP

Students: Pulling an all-nighter is less effective than studying and getting a good night's rest, as sleep helps cement learning and memory!

Sleep's effect on short- and long-term memory storage

Neuroscientists have found that sleep helps transfer memories and newly learned skills to a more long-term storage location in the brain's cortex. This transfer frees up space in the hippocampus for learning new information or skills the following day.

This transfer process from short- to long-term storage is facilitated by sleep spindles, the spikey bursts of brain activity occurring in N2 sleep. The more sleep spindles you fire off, the better your brain is at consolidating new memories and resetting for the next day's learning tasks.

The waves of brain activity during sleep also help sort and sift through older memories, including places you've been and people you've met. Imagine that your brain has an internal GPS that keeps track of all the places you've been. When you're asleep your brain reactivates and traces over these paths again. This makes it easier to find your way around your memories when you wake up.

TECHNICAL
STUFF

THE GLYMPHATIC SYSTEM AND ITS 2024 UPDATE

Since its discovery in 2013, the glymphatic system — combining "glia" and "lymphatic" — was thought to play a critical role in clearing away waste during sleep. It was believed to facilitate the removal of soluble proteins and metabolites from the brain, helping prevent conditions like Alzheimer's disease, with cerebrospinal fluid (CSF) flow through the brain's perivascular spaces being most active during non-rapid-eye-movement (NREM) sleep.

However, a 2024 study by Miao and colleagues in *Nature Neuroscience* challenged this understanding. Their findings showed that brain clearance is actually enhanced during wakefulness, not sleep. They measured clearance in mice and found it decreased during sleep and anesthesia, which contradicts the prior belief that sleep is essential for cleaning the brain.

Tuning Into Your Circadian Rhythms

Most people are aware that during the day, you naturally feel varying degrees of alertness and tiredness. Two main systems regulate wake and sleep.

>> **Sleep drive** builds throughout the day, driven by the accumulation of adenosine, which makes you feel progressively sleepier the longer you're awake.

>> **Your circadian clock,** influenced by the light-dark cycle, regulates sleep timing by releasing melatonin as night approaches, signaling your body to wind down for sleep.

Together, these two systems create the ebb and flow of sleepiness and alertness you experience daily. They ensure that you not only fall asleep but also stay asleep long enough to reap the restorative benefits. Understanding how these systems work can help you optimize your sleep patterns and brain health.

Mastering sleep drivers: Adenosine and alertness

One of the reasons you eventually fall asleep is because it becomes almost impossible to resist! The longer you stay awake, the sleepier you become due to rising sleep pressure.

Sleep drive is driven by adenosine

Your sleep drive system involves adenosine, a byproduct of ATP (your neurons' primary energy molecule). The longer you stay awake, the more adenosine levels build up in your brain, creating sleep pressure or the urge to sleep. Think of adenosine as a chemical stopwatch ticking away, telling you it's time for slumber after you've been awake for about 16 hours if you're a healthy adult.

As adenosine levels rise, they inhibit neuronal activity by locking into post-synaptic adenosine receptors. Activation of these receptors makes you feel sleepy, signaling that it's time to rest.

Caffeine blocks adenosine

Caffeine is the nemesis of adenosine! Caffeine operates as an adenosine receptor antagonist, meaning it binds to the same receptors in the brain that adenosine would. By attaching itself to these neural docking stations, caffeine prevents adenosine from exerting its usual sleep-inducing effects. Instead, caffeine ramps up neuronal firing.

So, next time you find yourself reaching for that afternoon coffee, remember it's caffeine waging war against your natural sleep pressure, keeping drowsiness at bay and your mind sharp. Now you know exactly why that cup of joe works its magic!

Setting your circadian clock

Understanding how to set your circadian clock can improve your sleep and overall health. Your internal timekeepers, known as clock genes, help align your biological rhythms with the 24-hour day.

Clock genes are internal timekeepers

Planet Earth spins on its axis every 24 hours. This rotation influences our biology, regulating key processes like blood pressure, body temperature, and sleep cycles. This daily rhythm is governed by clock genes found in nearly all cells, which align with the natural day-night cycle through environmental cues, or zeitgebers, like light and temperature.

The suprachiasmatic nucleus (SCN) in the hypothalamus acts as the master clock, using light and dark signals to sync your biological clocks with the day-night cycle. As night falls, the pineal gland secretes melatonin, signaling the body to prepare for sleep and keeping your internal rhythms in harmony with the natural world.

Other cues such as temperature and food timing (when you eat) also play a crucial role in aligning circadian rhythms to the 24-hour day.

Sunrise and sunset

Visual systems neuroscience research has recently shed light (joke!) on the crucial role of sunrise and sunset as zeitgebers. At sunrise, the sky transitions from the dark blues of night to the soft pinks and oranges of dawn. Similarly, at sunset, the colors shift from the bright yellows and oranges of daylight to the deep purples and blues of twilight. These color changes are *zeitgebers!* It turns out specialized retinal cells in your eyes detect the color shifts of dawn and dusk, helping to sync your internal rhythms with the external environment.

So, when you witness a beautiful sunrise or sunset, remember that it's not just a visual treat — it's your body's natural way of keeping time.

REMEMBER

Temperature regulation

As any pregnant or menopausal woman will tell you, body temperature and sleep are close sleeping buddies. Fluctuations in body temperature can significantly impact the quality of your sleep. When your body temperature is too high or too low, it can be challenging to fall asleep or stay asleep.

TECHNICAL STUFF

As night approaches, your core body temperature drops, aided by melatonin, which dilates blood vessels to release heat, especially through your hands and feet. It's the *cooling* that helps initiate sleep. Throughout the night, your temperature continues to fall, reaching its lowest point early in the morning before rising again as you wake. This temperature regulation is essential for maintaining and enhancing sleep.

Here are some tips to improve your sleep by tweaking your body or room temperature:

TIP

>> If you're struggling to sleep, try lowering the room temperature.

>> Taking a hot shower or using a sauna before bed, then cool off.

>> Ensure your bedding is suitable for the current temperature.

By adjusting your sleeping environment to facilitate heat loss, you can leverage your body's inherent rhythms to enhance sleep quality.

Adjusting the adolescent alarm

Adolescents often struggle with sleep schedules, and it's not just because they enjoy staying up late. At puberty their circadian rhythms naturally shift, making them want to go to bed later and wake up later. This phenomenon is known as *delayed sleep phase syndrome*.

TIP

Here are some tips to help your adolescent get the rest they need, despite their biological or social inclinations.

>> Try to get your teen up to see morning sunlight.

>> Reducing screen time before bed.

>> Establish a regular sleep.

>> Make your teen's bedroom conducive to sleep — cool, dark, and quiet.

Calculating your chronotype

Chronotypes are your body's natural preferences for wakefulness and sleep. In the science literature it's known as "morningness-eveningness" preference. They affect not only your sleep patterns but also your performance and activity levels throughout the day. Think of chronotype as whether you're an early bird or a night owl.

Your chronotype is largely genetic, with evidence suggesting a strong genetic component. Researchers use questionnaires such as the Morning-Eveningness Questionnaire (MEQ) and the Munich ChronoType Questionnaire (MCTQ) to categorize people's sleep preferences. One fun online quiz identifies chronotypes, categorizing people as bears, wolves, lions, or dolphins based on their sleep-wake patterns. I am a deep-sleeping lion — I wrote most of this book between 5 a.m. and 10 a.m., and I love to nap!

TIP

Understanding your chronotype can help you align your schedule with your natural tendencies, improving sleep quality and overall health.

Melatonin: The hormone of darkness

Melatonin, a hormone produced by the pineal gland, plays a critical role in regulating sleep-wake cycles. It is often called the "hormone of darkness" because its production ramps up as darkness falls. Its production increases in the absence of light (such as, after the sun goes down), signalling to the body that it's time to prepare for sleep. However, melatonin itself is not like a sleeping pill; instead, it sets the stage for sleep, acting as a "starter" rather than a participant in the sleep process.

TECHNICAL
STUFF

When light (sunlight or artificial light) hits your retina, it sends a signal to the suprachiasmatic nucleus (SCN) in your brain. The SCN is like the central pacemaker of your circadian clock and regulates most circadian rhythms in your body. In bright light, the SCN then sends messages via a neural pathway to the pineal gland, instructing it to suppress melatonin production. But when it's dark, the SCN allows the pineal gland to synthesize and release melatonin. This increase in melatonin levels signals to your body that it's time to prepare for sleep, making you feel drowsy as night approaches.

Melatonin has multiple actions within the body, many of which are linked to the regulation of circadian rhythms:

>> **Circadian and sleep regulation:** Melatonin signals night, promotes sleep onset, and synchronizes circadian rhythms with the light-dark cycle.

>> **Physical and hormonal effects:** It lowers core body temperature, affects hormone secretion (like reproductive hormones), and influences puberty and menstrual cycle.

>> **Antioxidant, immune, and cardioprotective functions:** Melatonin acts as an antioxidant, protects cells from free radicals, and may help lower blood pressure and reduce inflammation.

>> **Eye and gut health:** Melatonin protects eyes from damage (possibly reducing macular degeneration risk), promotes gut health, and supports digestion.

The effects of melatonin are complex and are mediated through interactions with specific melatonin receptors (MT1 and MT2) in the brain and other body tissues, as well as by its antioxidant action.

Melatonin supplementation for jetlag

Melatonin supplements are particularly helpful for adjusting your body's internal clock when dealing with jet lag, especially after crossing five or more time zones. It "tricks" your brain into aligning with the new time zone, making it an effective tool for preventing or reducing the effects of jet lag, such as when traveling long distances like from Sydney to San Diego.

Melatonin supplementation for children

Melatonin is often used to help children who have trouble falling or staying asleep. It can benefit children who are developing normally as well as those with ADHD, autism, other developmental disabilities, or visual impairments.

WARNING

Before considering melatonin as an easy fix, it's important to identify and address specific causes of children's sleep problems.

Melatonin supplementation if you just can't sleep

According to the Sleep Foundation, melatonin's main benefit is in reinforcing external cues for sleep or as a tool to help shift sleep-wake rhythms.

However, melatonin supplements aren't a magic fix for everyone, especially if you're not dealing with disruptions such as jet lag. The effectiveness of over-the-counter melatonin can vary, and regulations differ across countries regarding its sale. Also, don't underestimate the placebo effect —believing that melatonin will help you sleep can be surprisingly effective, harnessing the powerful mind-body connection!

Understanding the Consequences of Sleep Deprivation and Disruption

When you consistently miss out on quality sleep, it's not just about feeling tired. The consequences can be serious, affecting your emotional, cognitive, and physical health. Here's a quick overview of the effects of sleep deprivation, disruption or irregularity.

>> Skipping sleep can leave you feeling tired, moody, and more likely to get depressed.

>> Your stress response can go into overdrive, leaving you less resilient.

>> You might act impulsively, take risks, and your motor skills could suffer.

>> It becomes harder to focus and stay alert, making everyday tasks feel tougher.

>> Your memory takes a hit.

>> Decision-making slows down, which can be dangerous in high-risk workplaces.

>> Expect drowsiness, sudden microsleeps, and malaise.

>> Chronic lack of sleep can lead to serious health issues such as heart disease, cancer, diabetes, and metabolic problems

REMEMBER

In short, skipping out on sleep isn't just a minor inconvenience — it has serious repercussions for your emotional well-being, cognitive performance, and overall physical health.

Sleep and mood disorders

If you're dealing with depression, you may find yourself trapped in a cycle of troubling thoughts, irritability, difficulty concentrating, and a lack of energy. Poor sleep makes you feel worse. And these feelings worsen sleep. Many people with depression struggle to fall asleep, stay asleep, or feel excessively sleepy during the day. This means that poor sleep can contribute to the development of depression and having depression makes a person more likely to experience sleep troubles. Because the two are so closely related it can be a guessing game about which came first. It's a bit like asking, "What came first, the chicken or the egg?"

However, there's hope. By improving your sleep quality, you can better manage depressive symptoms, creating a more stable foundation for mental health.

Biological mechanisms linking sleep and mood disorders

According to the Sleep Foundation, about 40 percent of people with insomnia have clinical depression, and a whopping 80 percent of those with depression struggle with insomnia. The biological mechanisms underlying this link are complicated because sleep disturbance impacts the brain's regulation of mood through several pathways:

» Sleep disturbance disrupts the balance of neurotransmitters such as serotonin and dopamine, which are critical for mood regulation.

» Sleep disturbance activates the hypothalamic-pituitary-adrenal (HPA) axis, leading to heightened stress and anxiety.

» Inadequate sleep impairs synaptic plasticity and neurogenesis.

» Chronic sleep loss promotes inflammation.

Day and nightlight exposure

Your circadian rhythm and mood are intimate bedfellows. Circadian rhythm disturbances are a common feature in many mood disorders, highlighting the importance of these natural cycles in maintaining mental well-being.

Remember, daylight is the primary regulator of your circadian clock. This makes light exposure, the timing of that exposure or lack thereof a significant factor in psychiatric disorders. A fascinating study published in 2022 examined the connection between mental health and light exposure in 86,772 adults. The researchers concluded:

» Exposure to artificial light at night-time significantly increased the risk of psychiatric disorders, as well as poorer self-reported mood and well-being.

» Exposure to daylight during daytime reduced risk of psychiatric disorders, as well as better self-reported mood and well-being.

TIP

To improve and protect your mental health, it's crucial to get plenty of bright light (ideally natural sunlight) during the daytime and minimize your exposure to artificial light at night.

Sleep and cognitive function

Neuroscience and sleep science researchers have repeatedly highlighted how crucial adequate sleep is for maintaining cognitive performance. When you skimp on sleep, suffer insomnia, or do shiftwork, it doesn't just make you feel groggy; it tangibly affects your ability to concentrate, remember information, and make sound decisions. And staying awake even on a single occasion for more than 24 hours leaves you with reduced reaction times, attention, memory, and decision-making. This makes something as simple as driving your car quite dangerous.

Fatigue is a closely related problem. Fatigue is defined as a state of exhaustion that results from prolonged periods of wakefulness, high workloads, health issues, or lifestyle factors. It's driven by two main biological forces: Your homeostatic drive for sleep and your circadian rhythm.

REMEMBER

Essentially, your brain needs the right dose of sleep taken at the right time to function optimally, and when you don't get enough, it leads to excessive sleepiness — a major safety concern in many professions.

The impact of fatigue on workplace safety

Healthcare workers, including doctors, nurses, pilots, and cabin crew, often face long shifts and irregular hours, leading to significant sleep deprivation. Studies show that this lack of sleep can cause errors, putting themselves and others at risk, similar to the effects of being legally drunk. Airline staff, especially on ultra long-haul flights, also struggle with circadian rhythm disruptions, impairing cognitive functions and reaction times.

TIP

Prioritizing sleep isn't just about rest — it's a critical safety measure that sharpens your minds and safeguards your workplaces from costly mistakes.

Sleep and learning in the classroom

When it comes to classroom learning, sleep is just as critical for children and teenagers as it is for healthcare workers and pilots.

Insufficient, age-appropriate sleep quickly degrades children's ability to pay attention, learn, and play. Their capacity to absorb and learn new information hinges on their attention: Focusing on relevant information and filtering out distractions. Sleep not only helps you remember things but also enhances creativity and problem-solving skills, both essential for learning. When students get enough rest, they are better able to tackle difficult mental tasks, actively participate in class, and regulate their emotions.

TIP

So, whether you're clocking in for work or hitting the books, remember that a good night's sleep is one of your best tools for success.

Sleep and metabolic health

Sleep is also crucial for your metabolic health. And as discussed in various chapters in this book, brain health depends on metabolic health. And sleep is a crucial ingredient in the metabolic well-being recipe. How well you sleep can impact on your body's ability to maintain a healthy weight, regulate your blood sugar, and keep your heart healthy.

The relationship between sleep and metabolic health

Inadequate sleep — whether it's too short, too fragmented, or just poor quality — disrupts your body's metabolic processes. Metabolic syndrome a cluster of diseases characterized by abdominal obesity, high blood pressure, high triglycerides, low HDL cholesterol, and elevated blood sugar, is a major risk factor for cardiovascular disease and type 2 diabetes.

The link between sleep and metabolic health is a vicious cycle, where poor sleep contributes to hormonal imbalances, insulin resistance, and increased inflammation, all of which can lead to metabolic disorders. For example, inadequate sleep affects hormones regulating hunger and satiety (ghrelin and leptin), making overeating and weight gain more likely, while also impairing the body's ability to regulate blood sugar.

Snoring, sleep apnea, and metabolic syndrome

Snoring (which you've probably heard at some point!) is the noisy breathing during sleep caused by vibrating tissues. It's usually a harmless nuisance, mostly for the person lying awake next to the snorer! However, *obstructive sleep apnea* (OSA) is more serious. OSA involves repeated episodes of blocked airflow during sleep and is often a symptom of metabolic syndrome, highlighting how interconnected these health issues are.

This connection has led some experts to suggest renaming metabolic syndrome to *syndrome Z* to emphasize the role of sleep apnea. The same underlying issues, such as insulin resistance and excess visceral fat, drive both conditions, creating a dangerous cycle that heightens cardiovascular risks.

Obstructive sleep apnea (OSA), contributes to cardiovascular disease through several mechanisms like intermittent hypoxia, oxidative stress, and inflammation, raising the chances of heart disease and stroke. Frequent awakenings also boost sympathetic nervous system activity, elevating blood pressure and heart rate.

Ensuring you get enough high-quality sleep can help regulate your metabolism, keep your weight in check, and reduce your risk of chronic diseases.

Building Better Bedtime Habits

Everyone's sleep needs are different, but if you feel alert and functional during the day, you're likely getting enough sleep, even if it's less than the average seven to eight hours.

Sleep regularity versus sleep duration

In 2023, a fascinating study published in the journal *Sleep* shows the importance of getting to bed and waking up at regular times. The researchers analyzed over 10 million hours of accelerometer (a wrist movement tracker) data from 60,977 participants in the U.K. Biobank. They discovered that not just the duration, but the consistency of your bedtime and wake time may be an even more crucial predictor of health outcomes. They found that higher sleep regularity significantly lowered the risk of death from all causes, including cancer and cardiometabolic diseases.

TIP

What this means for you is that maintaining a consistent sleep schedule can be more beneficial for your health than just focusing on how many hours you sleep. So, for better health and a longer life, try to go to bed and wake up at the same time every day.

Perceiving what's healthy and normal

How you perceive your sleep quality can be skewed by the number of brief awakenings you experience.

It's perfectly normal for adults to wake up a few times during the night, usually during their lighter sleep stages. These awakenings are often so brief that you don't even remember them the next day. However, if you're prone to insomnia, waking up can trigger anxiety about falling back asleep, prolonging the wakeful period and worsening the insomnia.

Sometimes, waking from light sleep can feel like you've been awake for a while because your thoughts during light sleep mimic those we have while awake and relaxed in bed. People with insomnia often misjudge these awakenings, thinking they've been awake much longer than they actually have. A useful trick to differentiate between sleep and wakefulness is to check your memory — if you only have fragmented thoughts, you've likely just woken up; if you can recall detailed thoughts and worries, you've been awake.

Power Napping

Many people (me included!) have a strong natural inclination to nap in the afternoon. If you enjoy a regular power nap, or live where siestas are common cultural practice, you'll know how refreshed you feel after.

Some people sleep in the afternoon because they're catching up on missed sleep or they're unwell. Keep in mind that napping longer than one hour means you'll need less sleep that night because you'll have bumped adenosine off its receptors and reduced your sleep drive. My tip is to set an alarm for 20 minutes, so your power nap doesn't mess with your nighttime sleep.

Promoting a good sleep routine

Now that you understand how sleep works, you need to work on creating a sleep-friendly routine. A consistent day/night routine helps maintain regular sleep patterns.

TIP

Here are some tips to build a solid sleep routine:

>> **Daytime:** Maintain regular schedules for meals, medications, and activities to keep your body in rhythm. Morning sunlight is essential to sync your body clock, and regular exercise during the day will promote deeper sleep at night, but avoid long naps.

>> **Evening:** Avoid caffeine at least five hours before bed and opt for lighter meals if you're eating close to bedtime. Spend your last hour doing relaxing activities in dim light, and make your bedroom a comfortable, quiet, and cool environment.

>> **Bedtime:** Develop a calming bedtime ritual like taking a warm bath or brushing your hair, and only head to bed when you feel sleepy. Try to go to bed at the same time every night.

>> **Morning:** Wake up at the same time every day, regardless of how well you slept, and allow yourself time to fully wake up before evaluating how well you slept. And get some morning sunlight.

By following these tips, you can be well on your way to better sleep and a healthier life.

Overcoming Insomnia

Insomnia is a sleep disorder that makes it difficult to fall or stay asleep, which can negatively impact your next day and trigger various health issues. If you have insomnia, you may wake up too early and find it hard to fall back asleep. While most adults need seven to nine hours of sleep, many of us have experienced short-term insomnia due to stress or upsetting events.

Insomnia can be the main issue or a side effect of other problems. Chronic insomnia often stems from stress, life events, or health problems that mess with sleep.

As always, your first port of call for any health concern should be your family doctor or GP. Sleep science and insomnia treatment is a well-researched health-care issue and there are plenty of options to help you catch those elusive "Zs"!

Depending on the causes of your sleep problems, your doctor may recommend cognitive behavioral therapy, medications, other lifestyle inventions, or all the above.

Trying cognitive behavioral therapy for insomnia

Cognitive behavioral therapy for insomnia (CBT-I) is a structured, evidence-based approach to treating chronic insomnia. It helps you control or eliminate negative thoughts and behaviors that keep you awake. It's often the first line of treatment for insomnia and can be as effective, if not more so, than medication. Here's what it involves:

>> **Stimulus control therapy:** Set regular bed and wake times, avoid naps, and use the bed only for sleep and sex.

>> **Relaxation methods:** Techniques such as progressive muscle relaxation, biofeedback, and breathing exercises help reduce bedtime anxiety.

>> **Sleep restriction:** Limit time in bed to build sleep pressure and gradually increase it as sleep improves.

>> **Remaining passively awake:** Try to stay awake to reduce anxiety about falling asleep.

>> **Light therapy:** Use light exposure to shift your internal clock if you fall asleep or wake too early.

The only downside of CBT-I is it depends on trained clinicians, which can make it hard to access, expensive (depending on your healthcare system), and time-consuming. But there are some clever online apps such as Sleepio, SHUTi, and CBT-I Coach that are just as effective as a real human sleep clinician or coach!

Treating insomnia with pharmaceuticals

Treating insomnia often starts with CBT-I as the preferred approach, according to Australian guidelines. Medications may be used for short-term insomnia (under four weeks) to address underlying issues like stress or illness, but long-term use of sleep medications is not recommended beyond three months.

The choice of medication depends on the specific sleep issue. Quick-onset medications like temazepam or zolpidem help with falling asleep, while longer-acting medications such as nitrazepam are used for staying asleep but can cause next-day drowsiness. For circadian rhythm disruptions, melatonin may be helpful to reset the internal clock.

REMEMBER

It's important to be aware of potential side effects. Medications should be used cautiously and for short durations, with CBT-I being the long-term solution for managing insomnia.

Chapter **15**

Socializing Your Way to a Healthier Brain

From prehistoric campfires to family dinners, playgroups, schools, churches, restaurants, weddings, and funerals — humans gather. Maybe you watch your kids' sports games, cheer for Olympians, and sing along at concerts or in worship. These shared experiences don't just lift your spirits; they're a key to a healthy brain. Social engagement and relationships help maintain mental well-being, reduce your risk of dementia, and build resilience.

In this chapter you read about the neuroscience showing that strong social bonds aren't just a nice-to-have; they're essential for a healthy brain.

Understanding the Importance of Linked Lives

Human life is inherently social, with our most significant experiences and milestones deeply intertwined with those of others. This idea, called *linked lives*, stresses that people's lives are tied to and affect each other. Even though it's important, a lot of human development and neuroscience research has studied individual people in isolation and doesn't consider how important social relationships are.

I take this idea from a 2015 paper titled *Relationships in Time and the Life Course: The Significance of Linked Lives* by Richard A. Settersten, Jr. Settersten points out that your identities, opportunities, decisions, and the meanings you derive from life are all shaped by your relationships. Social connections play a crucial role in your life story, whether with individuals, groups, or communities.

The impact of social relationships on life's narrative

Setterson's observations about the power of social relationships in the life course may resonate with you. Here is my summary of his ideas:

>> **Your major life milestones often involve others.** Your life is influenced by events in the lives of those around you, and many life transitions bring new roles and relationships that affect not just you but also those close to you.

>> **You organize your life around others, negotiating and compromising on big decisions such as education, work, and family planning.** Maintaining relationships requires resolving conflicts and aligning your life with those of others.

>> **You gauge your life progress by comparing yourself to others, such as peers, parents at your age, or your future expectations.** These comparisons help you understand your experiences and milestones.

>> **Your identity is influenced by the people you associate with and aspire to be like.** Social experiences and interactions create your sense of self, resulting in multiple identities based on your relationships.

>> **Relationships can inspire you to achieve and persist.** For instance, as a first-generation college student (as I was), you may strive to succeed because your parents lacked such opportunities, or you may work to prove doubters wrong.

>> **Relationships can both stabilize and disrupt your life.** They can provide meaning and support but also pose risks and constraints. Relationships are key in transmitting advantages, disadvantages, and inequalities across generations.

Linking relationships to brain health

In your quest for better brain health, you become quite used to hearing about tips such as quitting smoking, cutting your alcohol intake, exercising regularly, and eating a balanced diet. These are vital and chapters in this book are devoted to them. But maybe you overlooked one of the most significant determinants of health: Social connectedness.

Underestimating the importance of social connections

Social relationships profoundly impact your mental and physical well-being, often surpassing the benefits of many traditional health behaviors. But despite robust evidence, people often underestimate the importance of social relationships for their health.

TECHNICAL STUFF

A survey of 500 individuals in the U.S. and U.K. asked respondents to rank various health factors. Social support was typically ranked last, even though meta-analyses show these factors are crucial predictors of mortality and more important than quitting smoking! This underestimation likely stems from the dominance of the biomedical model, which emphasizes biological and genetic determinants of health, overshadowing the equally significant social factors.

Defining social relationships

Before I take you through some examples of how social connectedness benefits brain health, it would be wise to define social connectedness. Here's a few different definitions in the literature so you can think more deeply about relationships and what they mean for brain health.

>> **Perceived social support** means you feel like other people care about you and are there for you. This definition puts more weight on how you feel about your support groups than how many you have.

>> **Social integration** involves your involvement in many social interactions, such as family, friends, and the community. It is often measured by how many and how often people communicate with each other.

>> **Belongingness** is about feeling accepted and valued within a group. This meaning stresses the emotional side of social ties and the need to feel like you belong.

>> **Network size and density** is a more quantitative and structural definition, focusing on network size and density, or the number of social connections a person has and how closely these relationships are linked. This way of measuring social closeness determines how big and how many connections you have in your social network.

>> **It's also important to understand the difference between being alone and loneliness.** Being alone, or *solitude*, is simply the physical state of being without others. On the other hand, *loneliness* is a negative emotion, where you feel empty and isolated, driven by your perceived lack of social connection.

All these different meanings show how complicated social connectedness is, showing how different parts of it affect a person's health and well-being as a whole. To study how social links affect health, understanding these subtleties is important.

The importance of attachment and the impact of neglect on brain health

Social relationships are foundational in infancy and childhood brain development.

Attachment theory is a psychological theory that stresses how important it is for kids to form warm, loving bonds with their carers early in infancy. This idea suggests that children who have what are called *secure attachments* — sensitive and emotionally available relationships — develop mentally and emotionally in a healthy way.

According to research in developmental neuroscience, these kinds of secure bonds are linked to better stress management, learning skills, and mental health in adulthood. These early social connections help mature brain networks that help control emotions and understand social situations. This sets the stage for lifelong mental health and well-being.

WARNING

Sadly, much of what we know about brain health and early childhood relationships comes from studies of neglect and trauma. Children who lack secure attachments in infancy and early childhood display significant cognitive and emotional deficits, underscoring the critical role that early social interactions play in healthy brain development. Such findings highlight the profound impact of secure attachments and nurturing environments on a child's future well-being.

How babies drive us to connect with them

Human babies come into the world with a fundamental biological need to be loved and comforted, and they are remarkably adept at communicating their needs without using words. Before a baby can make eye contact, smile, or use words to express their needs they use their two powerful tools to help new parents navigate the caregiving learning curve. Crying is one of their most effective communication methods. The other method is their adorable little face.

REMEMBER

Most mammals, including primates and humans, have irresistibly cute babies. If you were to draw an adorable baby bunny, puppy, kitten, or human, you'd likely include features such as big eyes, a button nose, round cheeks, a high forehead, and a chubby, squishy little body.

In academic literature, cuteness is often called *Kindchenschema*, a term coined by Austrian Nobel Prize winner Konrad Lorenz. He suggested that cuteness acts as an "innate releasing mechanism" for instinctual caregiving behaviors. Kindchenschema has since been expanded to include "auditory cuteness" such as high-pitched baby giggles and babbles, and "olfactory cuteness" such as the indescribably delightful smell of a baby (a scent so captivating that I once delayed bathing my second son for a week to enjoy it).

THE LONG-TERM EFFECTS OF EMOTIONAL NEGLECT

You may sadly remember the tragic stories from Romania in the late 1980s after the fall of Communist dictator Nicolae Ceausescu. Thousands of children were discovered in orphanages, suffering from severe malnutrition and social and emotional neglect. British families adopted many of these children, and researchers have tracked their progress, comparing them to U.K. adoptees who did not experience such deprivation. A significant study published in *The Lancet* in 2017 followed 165 Romanian adoptees, now in their mid-twenties. The findings revealed that Romanian adoptees had higher rates of low educational achievement, unemployment, and mental health issues, including depression and anxiety that began in their teenage years. They also displayed problems with attention, disinhibited social engagement, and autism symptoms. Notably, children who spent less than six months in the orphanages showed outcomes similar to U.K. adoptees.

The study concluded that severe adversity from early institutional deprivation can have long-lasting psychological effects, despite being later raised in nurturing and supportive environments. This research underscores the crucial importance of warm, nurturing relationships in early childhood for healthy brain development.

Human brains, regardless of sex or parental status, strongly prefer Kindchenschema. Cuteness triggers a swift and decisive response in the brain networks associated with motivation, pleasure, wanting, and liking. This neural prompt motivates us to engage in a more complex choreography of slow, careful, deliberate, and long-lasting prosocial behaviors to care for the baby.

Studying the Social Brain

Humans are social mammals who need neural systems to support social behaviors for survival and thriving.

Perceiving, processing, and relating: Three stages of social cognition

Understanding social cognition before learning about the social brain structure is important because it gives you a picture of how your brain processes and understands social information.

In social neuroscience, there are three stages of social information processing. Typically, the focus is on the middle one — cognition — but looking at all three stages is helpful to get a complete picture.

>> **Initially, you use your senses to perceive social information.** This means you quickly distinguish human from non-human entities through cues such as smell, touch, facial recognition, and speech. This stage is innate and immediate, happening almost without you realizing it.

>> **The second stage is social cognition.** This stage is where your brain works to understand others' emotions and intentions. You decipher feelings, plans, and affiliations using various brain networks. This process is swift and automatic, influenced by context, inference, and bias. Social neuroscience has pinpointed specific brain structures that activate more when considering others than nonsocial objects.

>> **Finally, the third stage involves regulating and controlling your responses in social situations.** This is where emotions are learned, controlled, and recognized, particularly those unique to social contexts. These emotions play a crucial role in how you interact with others. Individual responses in this stage can vary widely, and disturbances in this process can be observed in conditions such as autism or depression.

TIP

To make this more relatable, imagine a mom and daughter interacting after the girl comes home from school. The girl is feeling left out by her friends.

>> **At the perception stage,** the mother notices subtle cues in her daughter's voice, eyes, and body language. She picks up on the tone of voice, hesitations, eye contact, and posture. These are the mom's sensory perceptions.

>> **Next, in the cognition stage,** the mother pieces together these subtle cues. She reflects on what she knows about her daughter's life and concludes that her daughter may be feeling sad and lonely.

>> **Finally, at the behavior stage,** the mother responds to her perceptions and cognitions. She reaches out and gives her daughter a comforting hug and a few gentle words of encouragement. This behavior signifies understanding, support, and love. The hug is a way of communicating that she's there for her daughter and recognizes her feelings.

By understanding these three stages — perception, cognition, and behavior — you gain insight into the complex processes of the social brain and how crucial these processes are in everyday interactions.

How the social brain works

Over the past two decades, researchers have identified specialized brain regions that are consistently engaged during social, perception, cognition, and behavior. This is how your brain processes, understands and responds to other people.

Social brain networks

The social brain is made up of several networks, each with distinct roles (see Figure 15-1):

>> The amygdala-centered network detects social importance or *salience,* helping you respond to emotions such as fear, excitement, or affection. It enables you to connect with others by processing social cues.

>> The mentalizing network helps you understand what others may be thinking.

>> The empathy network helps process information on how you feel and understand others' emotions.

>> The action observation network activates when you watch others' actions and emotional expressions. It helps you understand and imitate their behaviors, which is crucial for learning social cues.

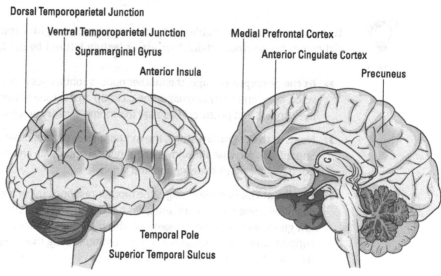

FIGURE 15-1:
Social brain
networks.

Dorsal Temporoparietal Junction
Ventral Temporoparietal Junction
Supramarginal Gyrus
Anterior Insula
Medial Prefrontal Cortex
Anterior Cingulate Cortex
Precuneus
Temporal Pole
Superior Temporal Sulcus

© John Wiley & Sons, Inc.

Key regions involved in these various social brain networks include:

>> Temporoparietal Junction (TPJ)

>> Dorsomedial Prefrontal Cortex (dMPFC)

>> Superior Temporal Sulcus/Gyrus (STS/STG)

>> Fusiform Face Area (FFA)

>> Ventromedial Prefrontal Cortex/Orbitofrontal Cortex (vMPFC/OFC)

Mirror neurons: Myth and reality

Mirror neurons have captivated many people with claims they're magic behind human empathy and social understanding, and people with autism have "broken" mirror neurons.

Mirror neurons make intuitive sense. Discovered in primates, mirror neurons activate when a primate performs an action and when that primate observes the same action being performed by another. This finding led to the hype that mirror neurons are the brain basis of human empathy, compassion, and understanding others' intentions.

WARNING

However, newer research has shown that this view is oversimplified and overdramatized. While mirror neurons help integrate sensory and motor information — such as when monkeys see and mimic each other's movements — they don't account for the full complexity of human social behaviors. Mirror neurons alone can't read minds or explain empathy, and they're not "broken" in people with autism.

Neuroscientists now refer to broader concepts such as the *action observation network* to explain these brain mechanisms. This network, rather than mirror neurons alone, is a smarter way to understand the brain's role in social behavior and relationships. Your social brain is far more complex and adaptable than once thought.

Thinking about others: Theory of Mind and Empathy

Understanding how you connect with and understand other people is fundamental to navigating social interactions. Two key concepts that help explain these social skills are Theory of Mind (ToM) and empathy.

Theory of Mind

ToM is your cognitive ability to understand that other people have their own thoughts, beliefs, intentions, desires, emotions, and knowledge, which can be different from your own. This skill is crucial for predicting and interpreting the behavior of others.

TIP

Imagine you see a friend looking around for their keys in the kitchen because they believe that's where they left them, even though *you* know the keys are actually in the living room. Your understanding of their belief, even if it's incorrect, is an example of ToM in action.

The development of ToM begins in early childhood. Around age two, children recognize that other people also have wants, needs, and feelings. By age three, many children understand that others can have different beliefs or thoughts, even if those beliefs are false. However, it's around age four to five that children can predict that others will act based on their false beliefs, marking a significant milestone in ToM development.

TIP

For example, imagine a five-year-old who knows their brother saw a toy under the bed, but later Mom moved it to a closet without their brother knowing. The five-year-old understands that their brother will look under the bed for the toy because that's where the brother last saw it.

Empathy

Empathy is your capacity to understand and resonate with another person's feelings, emotions, and perspectives. Empathy has both emotional (affective) and cognitive components.

>> **Affective empathy** is the feelings and sensations *you* experience in response to someone else's emotions. For example, if you see your son secretly wiping away tears because he didn't get picked for the team, you feel the pain of rejection as if it's your own. This immediate emotional response helps you connect with others and often motivates you to offer comfort or help.

>> **Cognitive empathy,** however, is your ability to understand and comprehend someone else's feelings and emotions. It's more about "thinking" than "feeling." Cognitive empathy enables you to understand someone else's perspective or point of view, even if you don't share the same emotions. For example, you may understand why your friend is frustrated with a tough deadline at work, even if you don't *feel* frustrated yourself. This kind of empathy is crucial for effective communication and problem-solving in social interactions.

When does empathy develop? Even newborns display a basic form of empathy called *emotional contagion* — for instance, hearing another baby cry may make them cry, too. As toddlers, children begin to show more affective empathy — recognizing distress in others and often trying to comfort them, such as hugging a crying friend. By preschool age, cognitive empathy starts to emerge, enabling children to understand that others have different feelings and perspectives from their own. Empathy continues to develop through middle childhood and adolescence, but life experiences and social and cultural norms in adulthood may shape how empathy is expressed.

The concept of "second-person neuroscience" and its implications

Human beings are social beings. But for decades, neuroscientists have studied human social brain networks in what I like to say is solitary confinement! We'd never dream of studying fish out of water, bees living alone away from their hive, or lions hunting antelope in a cage in the zoo. But, rather strangely, *other people* have largely been absent from social neuroscience.

Studying the human brain in social isolation

To help understand the social brain, the lone volunteer traditionally lies motionless inside a brain scanner. Inside the tightly confined space, they're shown photos, videos, or audio recordings of other people, or they're asked to (without moving) report on the mental or emotional state of the people they're watching on screen. All the while, their brain activity is monitored and analyzed to gain neural perspective of social relationships. While this traditional neuroscience research has provided many insights into the social brain; it's very different from studying how humans and their brains interact in the "wild."

Studying the human brain in real life interactions

While fMRI is excellent at showing *where* in the brain something happens, EEG shows precisely *when* something in the brain occurs. EEG has several additional benefits: It allows people to move around, have conversations, and experience other people in real-world settings. Most excitingly for social neuroscientists, EEG recordings can be made from two brains simultaneously.

This is such a new field of research that no one has quite yet landed on a shared vocabulary, so this method goes by various terms such as *dual-EEG*, *hyper-scanning*, or *second-person neuroscience*.

Neuroscientists are having a lot of fun using dual-EEG to show that when two people move their bodies in time, pay attention to the same book or movie, or have a conversation, their brainwaves also line up.

Here are some fun examples of dual-EEG research studies:

>> Researchers found that when two people move their bodies in sync, such as tapping their fingers together, their brainwaves also align. This interbrain synchrony suggests a neural basis for coordinated actions.

>> Studies involving cooperative games such as Jenga or solving puzzles together showed significant brain synchrony in the PFC.

>> During interactive teaching sessions, teachers and students exhibited synchronized brain activity in the temporoparietal regions. This neural alignment could play a role in effective learning and knowledge transfer.

>> When pairs engaged in creative tasks, such as brainstorming or joint drawing, their brain activity synchronized, particularly in areas associated with cognitive flexibility and problem-solving.

>> In experiments with violinists playing duets, researchers observed interbrain synchrony, emphasizing how music and rhythm can create deep neural connections between individuals. This synchrony extends to singing and other musical collaborations.

It's not ESP: How do two brains connect?

Bio-behavioral synchrony refers to the coordination or alignment of physiological and behavioral processes between two individuals, especially during social interactions.

This concept is often studied in close relationships between parents and their children. For example, when a mother and her infant engage in mutual gaze or share a playful moment, their behaviors align, and their physiological responses, such as heart rate or hormonal release, also become synchronized. Synchrony is believed to play a crucial role in social bonding, emotional regulation, and developing social skills and empathy, highlighting the deep interconnection between biological and behavioral responses in human relationships.

Bio-behavioral synchrony includes coordination of:

» Heart rate and breathing rate

» Pupil dilation

» Autonomic arousal

» Hormone release (for example, cortisol)

» Body movements

» Emotional experiences

» Brain waves (EEG)

Several mechanisms facilitate bio-behavioral synchrony: Eye gaze, shared body movements, body odor, and shared attention:

» Eye gaze signals intent and attention, leading to synchronized neural activity between two people.

» Moving in sync with another person, such as marching in time, tapping out a beat, dancing, or playing a sport.

» Body odor can trigger strong physiological and emotional responses, promoting bonding and synchrony.

» Sharing attention on the same object or activity, such as reading a book together or watching a movie.

CAN OUR BRAINS SYNC UP ON A ZOOM CALL?

Bio-behavioral synchrony can be significantly diminished during interactions via screens compared to face-to-face interactions. For instance, in a dual-EEG study with mother-child pairs, live face-to-face interactions showed robust brain synchronization, especially in frontal and temporal brain areas. However, when the pair chatted via a screen (similar to Zoom), this strong connectivity was greatly reduced, leaving only one significant link.

Even though social behaviors seemed similar, only live interactions had a clear relationship between brain activity and behavior. This suggests that face-to-face interactions involve unique brain processes that are not fully replicated through screens. Imagine replicating the deep connection of a shared laugh or a meaningful glance over a Zoom call — it doesn't have the same effect. This effect can be part of why you may feel "Zoom fatigue" after a day of virtual meetings, as the brain struggles with these limited connections, impacting overall communication and bonding.

Decoding the Biology of Love

Love is deeply rooted in your biology and affects every aspect of your life. It has inspired countless works of art and profoundly impacts your mental and physical well-being. A "broken heart" or failed relationship can lead to significant distress, and grief can disrupt your physiology, potentially leading to severe health consequences. People struggle to thrive without loving relationships, even if all other basic needs are met.

The oxytocin effect

When neurobiologists examine the anatomy and chemistry of love, they often focus on one molecule: oxytocin. Oxytocin, often called the "love hormone," plays a crucial role in social bonding, reproduction, and childbirth.

Oxytocin is a neuropeptide, a small protein used by neurons to communicate and is synthesized by neurons in the hypothalamus. It acts both as a neurotransmitter and a hormone. As a neurotransmitter, oxytocin influences brain regions involved in social and emotional processing, such as the amygdala, hippocampus, and nucleus accumbens. Once synthesized, it is also transported along axons to the pituitary gland, where it is stored in vesicles and released into the bloodstream as a hormone. This dual role enables oxytocin to impact various physiological and behavioral processes, making it integral to social interactions and emotional well-being.

Originally, oxytocin was primarily associated with its roles in labor and lactation. Early in the 1900s, British pharmacologist Henry Dale discovered that injecting pregnant cats with pituitary extract, which contained oxytocin, could hasten labor. This "hormone of swift birth" quickly found its way into human labor wards and is still used today in synthetic forms.

Oxytocin's role in mothering

Oxytocin is naturally produced, released, and regulated by your body during labor, delivery, and breastfeeding. It's responsible for uterine contractions during the third stage of labor when the placenta is expelled, and it continues to play a crucial role in milk let-down during breastfeeding.

Beyond its physical actions on smooth muscle, oxytocin helps establish a strong and lasting bond between you and your baby. This is why newborns are encouraged to breastfeed immediately after birth — the oxytocin released encourages uterine contractions, shrinking the womb, and reducing postpartum hemorrhage. One school of thought is that the hormones of pregnancy, birth, and breastfeeding prime birth mothers to focus intently on avoiding threats and thus keeping their baby alive.

The response to a crying baby

Research conducted by Bianca Jones Marlin, a neuroscientist at Columbia University has looked at how neurons adapt to motherhood, specifically how an existing social cue, such as a baby crying, gains relevance after pregnancy. She found that the hormone oxytocin is crucial.

In mice, the auditory cortex is rich in oxytocin receptors, and the presence of oxytocin, whether due to pregnancy or artificial introduction, rebalances neural activity. This rebalancing by oxytocin amplifies the ultrasonic distress calls of baby mice, enabling mother mice to respond to their pups' cries. Marlin speculated that a similar mechanism may make human mothers more responsive to their babies' cries when they breastfeed, as oxytocin is released during this process.

The "mama bear" response

The U.S. National Park Service advises "never place yourself between a mother bear and her cub or approach them." The chances of an attack escalate if she perceives you as a danger to her cubs. The term *mama bear* illustrates the protective instinct seen across species. Research shows that specific brain cells in mice become active during lactation to drive "lactation aggression" against threats.

Mama bear responses are consistent with what neuroscientists know about oxytocin — it enhances social cohesiveness and aggressiveness in humans and decreases stress and fear in animals. Numerous studies show lactating females are more resilient to electric shocks, looming predators, or being challenged to retrieve pups via a complex maze.

However, translating these animal findings to human maternal behavior (or your own feelings if you're a mom) is tricky, as human motherhood is influenced by social, psychological, and cultural factors. Unlike mice and bears, human mothers navigate complex emotional landscapes, social support systems, and personal experiences that also shape their responses to their babies.

Oxytocin and other relationships

Oxytocin is often talked about in terms of the special bond between a mother and her child, but it's also key in the connections between adults, especially in romantic relationships.

You probably never thought about prairie voles and titi monkeys before, but these are the darlings of oxytocin researchers because they're monogamous and endlessly loyal. Prairie voles, for example, pair up for life, and research shows that oxytocin and another hormone, vasopressin, play big roles in keeping these voles together. Titi monkeys are similar; they form close bonds with their partners, often seen cuddling with their tails intertwined, particularly under stress or while sleeping. This behavior is also linked to high levels of oxytocin receptors in their brains, emphasizing how crucial this hormone is for their relationships.

Scientists study these animals because their bonding patterns are simpler and more predictable than ours, which makes it easier to see how hormones such as oxytocin work in their brains. For example, when scientists change how oxytocin acts in prairie vole's brains, these normally faithful animals start acting more like their promiscuous relatives, the mice and rats. This shows just how powerful oxytocin can be in affecting behavior.

Oxytocin's role in stress reduction

Oxytocin may also be responsible for why social support protects against stress. Oxytocin makes you pro-social, encouraging you to seek social support when you're stressed. Oxytocin interacts with your stress-response and immune systems, reducing cortisol levels — a major stress hormone — in animals and humans. Oxytocin also has the following effects:

>> Reduces cortisol levels, mitigating the effects of stress.

>> Modulates the immune response, promoting healing and reducing inflammation. This effect is crucial in maintaining health during stressful periods, as chronic stress can lead to an overactive immune response and subsequent health issues.

>> Encourages social interaction creating a positive feedback loop. When individuals reach out for social support, their oxytocin levels increase, promoting social bonding and reducing stress. This loop can help explain phenomena such as forming strong bonds during shared traumatic experiences, where mutual support is critical for emotional and physical survival.

WARNING

However, translating from Titi monkeys or prairie vole's oxytocin levels to human relationships isn't straightforward! Your love life and how you connect with others are influenced by much more than biology. Humans have psychological aspects, such as your past experiences and your personality, and social factors, such as your culture and the expectations of those around you. While oxytocin plays a role in how you bond and connect with the people in your life, the full picture of human relationships is complex and influenced by more than the level of oxytocin in your bloodstream or synapses!

Confronting Loneliness and Its Health Implications

Loneliness isn't just about feeling sad; it's a health hazard. Being lonely is linked to premature death, and it can also lead to depression, high blood pressure, and even weaken your immune system. Similarly, those who are socially isolated are at increased risk of mental illnesses, emotional distress, and even dementia.

REMEMBER

Social isolation refers to having few social connections or infrequent contact with others. It's measurable and objective. Loneliness, however, is the *feeling* of being alone, regardless of the amount of social contact you have. It's subjective and about the quality, not the quantity, of your relationships.

>> **Loneliness:** When you feel unhappy because you don't have enough social connections or your relationships aren't fulfilling. It's a personal feeling of missing out on deeper, meaningful interactions.

>> **Social isolation:** This refers to the actual situation of having few social contacts or interactions. It's not just about feeling lonely; it's about not being socially active or having social support network.

The global loneliness epidemic

If you're feeling lonely, you're not alone. Loneliness is not just a personal issue; it's a significant global health threat. The World Health Organization (WHO) has recognized loneliness and social isolation as critical public health challenges that need urgent attention.

In 2023, the WHO established an international commission, led by notable figures including the U.S. Surgeon General, Dr. Vivek Murthy, and the African Union youth envoy, Chido Mpemba. The commission comprises advocates and government ministers from diverse backgrounds and regions, such as Vanuatu and Japan, to specifically focus on loneliness and isolation as a public health problem. The WHO statistics reveal that about one in four older adults globally experience social isolation, and loneliness affects between one in ten to one in five teenagers. These rates include low, middle, and high-income countries. The good news is that reports of loneliness among older folks (people 65 years and older) have been decreasing since 2001! This may be due to people over 65 being healthier and wealthier than past generations and prioritizing active social lives after retirement.

How the brain benefits from social interaction

Ever noticed how a juicy conversation or hooting laugh with friends can lift your spirits? Emotional support filled with empathy, love, and trust does wonders for your brain.

Imagine an elderly person — your Nan or your dad — who was once busy, working, connected to you and your family and full of life, now sitting alone day after day, with no visitors, no phone calls, and no one to share their thoughts or memories with. This stark reality is more common than you may think and highlights the heart-wrenching impact of social isolation.

Social connectedness and depression

When it comes to depression, one important but often overlooked contributing factor is social connectedness. Research shows over and over that loneliness is a strong risk factor for developing depression. Research in Europe and Japan has shown that older folks who feel lonely are significantly more likely to exhibit signs of depression, regardless of the number of social contacts they have. This highlights the profound impact of relationship quality and feelings of loneliness, not just lack of support, on mental health.

In contrast, women who lack social connectedness, especially and practical support during pregnancy and early motherhood experience higher rates of depression and anxiety compared to those with a caring partner or a supportive network of friends and family.

Social connectedness, brain aging, and dementia

Social connectedness also plays a vital role in protecting against cognitive decline and reducing the risk of dementia.

The 2020 Lancet Commission on dementia prevention estimated that tackling social isolation could prevent four percent of dementia cases worldwide, stating, "Good social connections (that is, living with others, weekly community group engagement, interacting weekly with family and friends, and never feeling lonely) are associated with slower cognitive decline."

Loneliness and social isolation are linked to poor health outcomes more broadly, increasing the risk of death from all causes, including cancer and cardiovascular disease. Overall, people with good social connections experience less cognitive deterioration as they age. This evidence underscores the importance of fostering strong, supportive relationships to enhance your mental health and protect your brain health as you age.

REMEMBER

Ultimately, no one should have to endure the profound loneliness that steals both years and joy from life. Understanding and addressing the importance of social connections can help ensure a healthier, happier, and longer life for yourself and those around you.

How loneliness impacts health

So now that you read that both social connections and loneliness influence health, you may now be wondering *how* loneliness gets under your skin and impacts your health? A few potential mechanisms are at play.

» **Neuroprotection:** You can think of social stimulation as an enriching intellectually stimulating experience — a topic I delve deeper into when we explore cognitive resilience in Chapter 17. Social interactions are cognitively challenging, potentially increasing cognitive reserve and resilience.

» **Stress reduction:** Strong, supportive relationships can help reduce stress and its physiological impacts, such as lowering blood pressure and improving immune function.

» **Social and emotional support networks:** People with active social lives are more likely to engage in healthy behaviors, such as exercising and following medical advice, due to shared norms and encouragement from peers. And people with strong social support networks have people to support with such as shopping, housework, and driving to medical appointments.

Conversely, loneliness and social isolation can have detrimental health effects.

THE CRUEL CYCLE OF POOR HEALTH AND ISOLATION

Imagine George, a 72-year-old gentleman who was once a beloved and active member of his neighborhood and a familiar face helping behind the scenes at community events. However, his life took a stark turn when he was diagnosed with Parkinson's disease. As the symptoms progressed, George found it increasingly difficult to maintain his busy lifestyle. Gradually, his community connections dwindled; friends visited less often, perhaps assuming he needed rest, and George's world grew smaller. This isolation worsened his health problems. Lacking practical support to attend medical appointments, George sometimes missed crucial check-ups and treatments. His diet suffered as he no longer had the energy to cook balanced meals or shop for groceries. As his condition deteriorated, he needed more support, but the diminishing social connections made accessing this help increasingly difficult. This isolation not only exacerbated his health issues but also deepened his loneliness and despair.

George's story (which I made up but feels painfully real) highlights the cruel cycle of poor health and isolation. By recognizing and tackling these challenges, we can better support individuals like George, ensuring they receive the essential care and social interaction needed to sustain their health and spirits.

Prescribing Social Connection and Support

Loneliness is heartbreaking. Feeling lonely can create a sense of social isolation, which often leads to a negative spiral. When loneliness sets in, it can become harder to reach out to others, making you feel even more disconnected.

TIP

You can take simple, practical steps to feel more connected and less isolated. And, for those who're curious about the scientific support for these tips, they've been tested out in real-world trials of lonely people. Here are some tips to help you, no matter your age:

>> **Find your people.** Make a list of all the people and groups you're already connected with, such as family, friends, workmates, or online communities. Recognizing who you already connect with is the first step.

>> **See who makes you happy.** Take time to think about which groups or friends make you happiest and most supported, and which leave you feeling flat or worse about yourself. Spend more time with those who lift you up.

>> **Try something new.** Look for new activities that interest you. Join a local book club, a gardening group, or a volunteer organization. If you're into

gaming, find an online gaming community. Trying something new can help you meet fresh faces.

» **Strengthen your bonds.** Spend more time with the people who matter. Schedule regular coffee dates, family dinners, or game nights with neighbors. Consistent interaction strengthens bonds.

» **Set social goals.** For example, aim to attend one new group activity a month. Use these group settings to practice starting conversations or offering help.

» **Check your social pulse.** Reflect on how your social activities make you feel. Keep a simple journal noting when you felt happiest and adjust your plans based on these reflections. Plan more outdoor activities if you felt great after a hike with friends.

» **Ask for advice.** Don't be afraid to ask for advice. Talk to a trusted friend, a family member, or a counselor about your social life. They can offer valuable insights and support.

» **Get involved.** Join in community activities. Volunteer at a local shelter, join a sports league, or participate in neighborhood events. If you're feeling isolated, sometimes a small step like calling a friend or attending a local fair can make a big difference.

» **Use social media smartly.** Engage actively on social media. Join groups related to your hobbies, participate in online discussions, and connect with like-minded people. Avoid passive scrolling, which can increase feelings of loneliness.

» **Get a pet.** Dogs, cats, or even smaller pets such as hamsters can provide great companionship and help reduce feelings of isolation. They're not just pets; they become part of your social network.

Taking these steps can help you build a more connected and fulfilling social life, reducing feelings of loneliness and improving your overall well-being. Remember, starting small and taking things one step at a time is okay.

IN THIS CHAPTER

» Understanding what's cognitively challenging

» Enriching your world with education and employment

» Interrogating the benefits of computerized brain training

» Peering into personality traits

» Finding your life purpose

Chapter **16**

Challenging Your Cognition for Better Brain Health

Understanding how to maintain and even enhance your cognitive abilities is crucial for healthy aging. This chapter explores how engaging in cognitive challenges can help build cognitive reserve, delay dementia onset, and promote overall brain health.

But maintaining cognitive function is not just about staving off dementia. It's about finding joy in the activities that engage your mind. Cognitive challenges are not merely tasks to keep your brain sharp but opportunities to discover new interests, deepen your knowledge, and connect with others. Whether it's learning a new language, picking up a musical instrument, or engaging in stimulating conversations, these activities can enrich your life and make every day feel as exciting and fulfilling as the "good old days."

Characterizing Cognitive Challenge

As you get older, your risk of cognitive decline and dementia increases. But remember none of this is inevitable, and the cognitive decline rate varies significantly from person to person.

Understanding cognitive reserve

Cognitive reserve is a phrase coined by neuroscientist Yakov Stern to explain your brain's ability to keep working well despite age-related changes or dementia-like pathology. It's like a buffer that allows you to continue functioning normally even as your brain undergoes the inevitable wear and tear of aging.

As you age, your brain naturally changes. Some people experience significant cognitive decline, while others remain sharp. This variation can be partly explained by cognitive reserve. Higher cognitive reserve can slow the onset of cognitive impairments and dementia, allowing you to maintain better cognitive function longer despite aging or brain pathology.

While brain reserve is relatively fixed, cognitive reserve can be enhanced by your experiences and activities throughout life.

Understanding memory: What it is and how it changes over time

Memory is a fundamental aspect of our identity and daily functioning. It is not just a passive storage system but an active, dynamic process that evolves over time.

Memory and aging

Some cognitive skills such as working memory and verbal fluency tend to decline with age. In contrast, others such as vocabulary and comprehension may even improve in midlife.

Most of the time, age-related cognitive changes aren't a major concern. But knowing the different aspects of memory and mental skills, and understanding what changes to expect as you age, is essential for distinguishing between normal aging and when it may be necessary to seek medical advice. The Alzheimer's Association has a great summary table outlining ten signs and symptoms of dementia with examples of normal aging for you to review.

Making meaning of your changing cognitive skills

Memory isn't just a record of your past; it's also important for being in the now and making plans. Neuroscientists now understand that your memory is not fixed but reshaped each time you recall an event. This continual reorganizing or reframing of a memory enables you to integrate new information and perspectives as you age.

I am a fan of the idea proposed by neuroscientist and memory researcher Dr. Charan Ranganath, who explains that as you age, your brain changes appropriately for your stage of life. He points out that in your younger years, your brain is highly goal-oriented, focusing on immediate tasks such as moving ahead in your career and building a family. However, as you grow older, your role evolves to take on a more collective function, enabling you to contribute meaningfully to your community and maintain a sense of purpose.

Examining cognitive reserve

To maintain cognitive health, it's essential to regularly engage in activities that challenge your mind.

Enriching your environment

At the turn of the century, while I was working towards my PhD, another research group from my department published a landmark study demonstrating how environmental enrichment can slow the progression of neurodegenerative diseases, specifically Huntington's Disease (HD) in mice.

Environmental enrichment means providing a busy and stimulating environment for lab mice that includes lots of sensory, cognitive, and motor activities (tunnels, wheels, boxes, and places to hide and play). Compared to HD mice kept in standard empty cages, HD mice living in enriched environments delayed the onset of HD symptoms. This extraordinary finding highlighted the crucial role of the environment in the progression of neurodegenerative diseases.

REMEMBER

Enriched environments are important for humans, too! One way to think about it is to consider the opposite way to live: staying in one room, sitting on the same chair, and watching the same episode of the same TV show hour after hour, day after day. Imagine the monotony of every day without ever trying something new.

Education and cognitive reserve

Education plays a key role in protecting your brain as you age. The Rotterdam Study was well-publicized research from the 1990s that was among the first to show that people with more years of formal education (school and college) were more resilient to brain aging. In short, more education helped maintain cognitive function for longer.

An international research study led by the Centre for Healthy Brain Ageing (CHeBA) at UNSW Sydney has found that more years of education can significantly decrease the risk of dementia. The study also highlighted that the protective association between higher education (attending college) and cognitive decline was stronger in women than men. Interestingly, it also found that people with different levels of education had similar brain pathology at death. In short, education helps you manage and compensate for brain changes more effectively.

Even if your school days are long behind you, it's never too late! Read, learn new skills, stay socially active, and challenge yourself mentally.

Employment and cognitive reserve

The complexity of your job also plays a crucial role in maintaining cognitive function as you enter your golden years.

Occupational complexity is an insightful way to measure the cognitive demands of your job. Occupational complexity involves working with people, data, or things, each requiring different mental abilities.

In another study, University of Michigan researchers gathered data from thousands of participants through questionnaires and interviews, asking them to report their main occupations and years spent working in each. The jobs were then coded into three complexity ratings: complexity of work with data, people, and things. Jobs were rated on a scale from zero (most complex) to eight (least complex), depending on the type of work. They found that jobs with greater mental demands, such as data analysis, strategy development, decision-making, and problem-solving, were linked to better cognitive functioning before retirement and slower memory decline after retirement.

Retirees who had worked in jobs with greater mental demands were more likely to have better memories before they retired, *and* more likely to have slower declines in memory *after* retiring than people who had worked in jobs with fewer mental demands.

Whether you're still working or long past retirement, seek out activities that challenge you mentally, whether learning new skills, engaging in creative hobbies, or solving complex problems. Your brain will thank you for it!

Building cognitive reserve

But what if you're decades past formal education or already retired? Enriching your environment is key to maintaining your cognitive reserve. It's not just about "mental activity" — think of it as keeping your brain lively and engaged with the world.

TIP

Keeping your mind sharp and engaged is essential for maintaining cognitive health as you age.

>> Join a book club.

>> Participate in community events such as choir or music groups.

>> Teach or mentor to share your knowledge and stay socially connected.

>> Travel and explore new places to experience different cultures and environments.

>> Pick up a new hobby such as knitting, woodworking, or painting.

>> Take a class or workshop on topics that interest you.

>> Stay involved in your field through part-time work, consulting, or volunteering.

>> Teach others informally to share your skills with friends and family.

>> Attend lectures and workshops to engage with new ideas and perspectives.

By incorporating these activities into your routine, you can create a rich, stimulating environment for your brain. Remember, it's not just about doing crossword puzzles — it's about engaging in various enjoyable and challenging activities that keep your mind, body, and social life vibrant. So go ahead, try something new, and keep your brain buzzing!

REMEMBER

Building and maintaining cognitive reserve is essential for healthy aging. Engaging in lifelong learning, pursuing meaningful and purposeful activities, and incorporating cognitive challenges into your daily life can enhance your brain health and reduce the risk of cognitive decline. Remember to combine mental challenges with social and physical activities for the best results. Stay curious, keep learning, and enjoy the journey of continuous mental growth.

EXAMPLES OF DIFFERENT COGNITIVE AGING TRAJECTORIES

Here's how the lives of three older men (not real people or names!), Albert, James, and Tom, illustrate for you three different cognitive aging trajectories.

First up we have **Albert,** a retired university professor of classics. He spent his life engaged in complex problem-solving and teaching. His extensive education and stimulating career built a robust cognitive reserve. He's now in his 80s and remains mentally agile, actively reading, and participating in academic discussions.

Next, we have **James,** who had a glamorous career as a luxury car salesman. While his job wasn't what you'd consider "intellectual," he needed to be good with people, negotiate, strategize, and know the latest trends in his field. All these factors kept his brain healthy. Even though James is retired, he still enjoys neighborhood events and keeps up-to-date with the car industry.

Finally, we have **Tom,** who worked in a factory assembling small parts on a production line for over 40 years. His job required him to do the same functions over and over again, with little room for change or problem-solving. Tom had a quiet life outside of work and didn't have many friends. Now that he's in his 80s, his cognitive loss is problematic. Because he doesn't have a lot of brain reserve, he is more likely to have memory and problem-solving problems as he ages.

Assessing the Effectiveness of Brain Training Programs

In today's tech-driven world, advancements in technology are revolutionizing healthcare, and brain health is no exception.

Testing the benefits of mental challenges and brain games

You may have encountered various brain training games on the market, promising to boost your memory, attention, and problem-solving skills. These games, while popular, offer mixed results. Studies show that they can improve the specific cognitive skills they target — if you're testing your verbal memory, you'll score better at sitting the verbal memory test — but they have *not* been proven to reduce the risk of dementia or treat AD.

Some companies have faced legal actions for making unsubstantiated claims about their computer games preventing dementia and now wisely make more cautious claims about general cognitive improvements.

Does computerized cognitive training (CCT) prevent brain aging?

When considering computerized cognitive training (CCT), research offers mixed results. A 2014 review of 52 randomized trials with nearly 5,000 participants found that CCT had small but statistically significant improvements in cognitive function. While it modestly improved nonverbal and working memory, it didn't impact executive function or attention.

The effectiveness of CCT depends on how it's done. Home-based programs were ineffective, while group-based training showed better results. Training more than three times a week or for under 30 minutes also didn't help. Structured, supervised group sessions seem to offer the most cognitive benefits for older adults.

Transferring virtual skills into real life

A significant question remains: Do the skills you develop via CCT transfer to real-life tasks?

Transference refers to the phenomenon where improvements in one cognitive domain lead to benefits in other untrained areas. For example, if a brain training game improves your verbal memory, are you better at remembering a list of words when you're not sitting at your computer?

Sadly, the evidence for such transference is limited for the types of CCT currently in use. While transference works well in simulated environments such as flight simulators, where the skills practiced directly mimic real-world tasks, it is less effective for individual cognitive skills.

The fact that CCT is not very transferable reveals one of the flaws inherent in brain training: Designing programs that improve specific skills and make real differences in everyday life.

Looking at the downsides of CCT

I personally am not too concerned with the limits of CCT. Even if it did "work," there is one major potential downside: The sedentary nature of CCT.

If you're still employed, have a busy social life, or read books on neuroscience and brain health, you're unlikely to need to spend time in front of a computer training your brain! Go for a walk instead.

Taking a smart approach to brain training

Just like with your diet and exercise regimen, it's crucial to be intentional, purposeful, and balanced with your digital activities.

>> **Intentional:** Be present and aware of your actions online.

>> **Purposeful:** Engage in activities that contribute to your goals and values.

>> **Balanced:** Limit screen time to maintain balance with physical and social activities.

Though CCT can offer some cognitive benefits, they are not a magic bullet for preventing cognitive decline or dementia. Incorporating an approach that includes physical exercise, social engagement, and a balanced relationship with technology is essential. This way, you can keep your brain healthy and enjoy a fulfilling, active life.

Seeking Purpose and Passion for Brain Health and Longevity

Purpose is the psychological tendency to derive meaning from life's experiences and possess a sense of intentionality and goal directedness. It sounds fluffy to talk about passion and purpose in a book about brain health, but the two are linked.

Peering in at your personality traits

Personality traits are well described in psychology, but harder to define from a neuroscience perspective. I like to think of them as patterns of thought, behavior, and emotion that are influenced by the brain's structure and function.

The Big Five

Personality traits are often described by using the Big Five personality traits. These traits are:

- **» Openness to experience:** Imaginative, curious, and open to new ideas

- **» Conscientiousness:** Organized, dependable, and goal-oriented

- **» Extraversion:** Sociable, assertive, and talkative

- **» Agreeableness:** Kind, cooperative, and compassionate

- **» Neuroticism:** Emotionally unstable, prone to anxiety and mood swings

These traits are widely studied in psychology and provide a comprehensive framework for understanding individual differences in personality and behavior.

Personality traits predict life satisfaction

A 2024 study of analysis explored how much personality traits influence overall life satisfaction. Using data from large groups in Estonia, Russia, and the U.K., researchers combined self-reports and reports from others to get a clear picture. They found that traits such as emotional stability (versus neuroticism) extraversion, and conscientiousness were strongly linked to being satisfied with life, while traits such as openness and agreeableness had a smaller impact.

Interestingly, people who often felt misunderstood, unexcited, indecisive, envious, or bored tended to have lower life satisfaction.

Purpose in life: Exploring the evidence

Conscientiousness, extraversion, and neuroticism have been linked to various health outcomes. For example, conscientious people — those who tend to be organized and responsible — typically engage in healthier lifestyles and have lower risks of cognitive decline. Extraverts — who are more social and outgoing — reap the benefits of stronger social networks that provide emotional support and mental stimulation. Whereas people with high levels of neuroticism — they're more anxious and emotionally unstable — have worse mental health.

You can see how personality traits' influence may directly affect our cognitive health and thus well-being.

Living a life on purpose

Some researchers have taken the brave step of quantifying how "on purpose" someone lives their life. Using a 10-item scale derived from Ryff's Scales of

Psychological Well-Being, they scored people as "high" or "low" in life purpose based on their answers to questions such as:

>> I feel good when I think of what I have done in the past and what I hope to do in the future.

>> I live life one day at a time and do not really think about the future.

>> I tend to focus on the present because the future nearly always brings me problems.

>> I have a sense of direction and purpose in life.

>> I enjoy making plans for the future and working them to a reality.

One study from the Rush Medical Center in Chicago, assessed over 900 older adults without dementia, evaluating their sense of purpose and tracking their cognitive health over up to seven years. They concluded having meaning and purpose in life can lower the risk of Alzheimer's disease and cognitive impairment as people age. Other health benefits linked to people who score high on life purpose include:

>> Better sleep

>> Happiness, satisfaction, and self-acceptance

>> Better mental health, less depression

>> Improved brain health, cognitive resilience, and longevity

Living purposefully in the blue zones

Let's be real, I know talk of "finding your purpose" can sometimes feel stressful or a bit lame, like a cheesy self-help meme. But there are plenty of useful tools to start exploring your purpose.

One is to think about the concept of *ikigai*, which translates to "reason for being" and is a central part of Japanese culture, especially in Okinawa, one of the world's *blue zones*. Blue zoners living in Costa Rica, refer to this sense of purpose as *plan de vida*. Or a much more pragmatic way to start is by considering your strengths by using the free VIA Strengths Finder tool online. This tool helps you identify your core strengths, providing a foundation for finding purpose.

Here are a few other tips inspired by blue zones:

>> **Do an internal inventory.** Reflect on your ideals, principles, standards, and morals. Consider your physical, emotional, and mental strengths. Write them

down and see what resonates deeply with you. Craft a Personal Purpose Statement based on these reflections.

>> **Put your skills into action.** If you discover a passion for something, such as animals, consider volunteering at a local shelter. Using your skills for good can bring immense satisfaction and health benefits, including lower rates of cancer, heart disease, and depression.

>> **Create a space for your passions.** Dedicate a spot in your home to display items that reflect your accomplishments and passions. This visual reminder can boost your sense of pride and purpose.

>> **Find a partner.** Share your life purpose and action plan with a trusted friend, family member, or colleague. Their feedback can help refine your plan and keep you motivated.

Ask yourself two key questions

To wrap up this section, I'd like to share with you my personal prescription for life purpose, using my strengths, and staying on track with my mental well-being. I ask myself two essential questions:

>> Is it awesome?

>> Does it help?

These questions help me align my daily actions with my deeper sense of purpose. Living with purpose can reduce stress, clarify your goals, and make you less dependent on others' opinions. It's about serving a cause bigger than yourself. Finding intrinsic meaning is crucial for a fulfilling life in a world increasingly driven by extrinsic values.

Prescribing Cognitive Challenges for Your Brain

Here's a list of fun, engaging, and motivational activities to help you stay mentally active:

>> **Join a walking book club.** Discussing books while walking with others can provide a mental and physical boost. My book club completes a 35km walk along our beaches every year!

>> **Participate in community theatre.** Whether you're acting, directing, or helping behind the scenes, it's a great way to stay engaged and connected with others.

>> **Teach a class or mentor.** Share your expertise by teaching a class or mentoring someone.

>> **Travel and explore.** Visit new places, whether near or far, to stimulate your brain with new experiences, cultures, and environments.

>> **Learn a new craft.** Pick up a hobby such as knitting, woodworking, or painting. Learning and mastering a new craft can be both relaxing and mentally stimulating.

>> **Take continuous learning courses.** Enroll in courses, workshops, or self-study programs on interesting topics. I teach online neuroscience and brain health courses — join me to learn!

>> **Stay mentally active in your field and teach others.** Even if you're retired, engaging in familiar yet challenging work can keep your cognitive skills sharp.

>> **Engage in thoughtful and purposeful computerized training if you choose to do so.**

REMEMBER

Focus on activities that bring you purpose, passion, and optimism to enrich your life and mind. And when evaluating activities, continue to ask yourself: Is it awesome, and does it help?

5

Avoiding Brain Health Hazards

IN THIS CHAPTER

» Defining stressors, stress responses and behaviors

» Exploring your physiological stress response systems

» Understanding the consequences of chronic or toxic stress

» Building resilience

» Finding your way to calm

Chapter 17

Buffering Against Toxic Stress

L ife is full of challenges, and I suspect you've managed to face many of them with remarkable resilience. It may not always feel that way, but the fact that you're here reading this book is evidence of your ability to thrive.

Your body's stress response systems help you deal with all sorts of threats, challenges, and opportunities that life throws at you. Stress is an essential neural and physiological response crucial for your survival. The issue with your stress response is that if it lasts too long, it can harm your brain and body, especially during critical periods in your life. Understanding how it works can help you better manage its effects.

Recognizing and Defining Stress

I don't like the word *stress*! Mostly because it lumps together everything from stressful *events* and physiological stress *responses* to the *feeling* of being stressed. This broad and vague usage makes it difficult to explore these distinct aspects in depth. So, I'm going to redefine them.

Defining stress, stressors, and feeling stressed

The term *stress* has evolved over time. Once upon a time it was used in the building and engineering disciplines where it referred to physical pressures on materials or structures. Now it's often used to describe a wide range of experiences and reactions, making it a challenging concept to explore deeply. To clarify our discussion, I differentiate between three key components: stressors, physiological stress responses, and subjective experiences or feelings of being stressed.

WARNING

By clearly distinguishing between stressors, physiological stress responses, and subjective experiences, we can better understand the complexity of stress. This differentiation enables us to explore each aspect in greater depth and develop more targeted strategies for managing stress.

Stressors

Stressors are external events or triggers that challenge you. Stressors can range from immediate threats to your safety, such as breaking a leg, to personal losses, such as losing a job or a loved one, to broader challenges such as global crises (who has quite yet recovered from the stressor of the pandemic). Understanding stressors is crucial because they are the initial triggers that set off your body's stress response.

Imagine facing a sudden job loss. This event is a *stressor* that can disrupt your life.

Physiological stress responses (neural and hormonal)

Once a stressor is present, your body and mind react through neural and hormonal pathways. This physiological *stress response* includes a range of reactions that prepare you to deal with the challenge. These responses can vary greatly among individuals.

TIP

When faced with a stressful situation such as an impending deadline, you may experience physical symptoms such as headaches or muscle tension, while someone else may feel anxious or irritable. These responses are your body's way of preparing to tackle the stressor.

Subjective experiences or feelings of stress

The subjective *experience of stress* is deeply personal and varies widely from person to person. It includes how you perceive and interpret stressors — will this help me or kill me? Your emotional reactions and the meaning you assign to your feelings play a crucial role in shaping your overall response to stress, influencing both your mental and physical health outcomes.

TIP

A breakup may be devastating for you, causing you to feel overwhelmed and stressed. For someone else, the same breakup may be seen as an opportunity for a fresh start and personal growth. These different reactions highlight the personal nature of stress experiences.

Understanding different types of stress

Based on our definitions, you can start to think about different types of stressors, different durations of stress responses, and whether the consequences are "good" or "bad."

>> **Physical:** Stressors like trauma, injury, or extreme temperatures that physically challenge the body.

>> **Psychological:** Mental challenges like exams or social embarrassment, whether real (an exam) or imagined (a monster under the bed!).

>> **Acute:** A brief, immediate response to threats (for example, avoiding a car accident) that triggers a rapid release of hormones, affecting future responses.

>> **Chronic:** Prolonged stress (for example, grief or caregiving) that lasts weeks or longer, often affecting mental health.

Sometimes, stress responses are framed in terms of your ability to cope with whatever challenge has come your way. Beyond acute, chronic, physical, and psychological, you may see the following definitions:

>> **Positive (eustress):** A motivating stress that enhances performance and builds resilience, often seen in positive challenges (e.g., starting school, preparing for sports competition).

>> **Distress:** Negative stress from perceived threats, leading to anxiety, poor performance, and physical/emotional symptoms, often tied to chronic stress.

Finally, stress responses, especially when discussed in the context of childhood experiences, are often framed as tolerable or toxic.

>> **Tolerable:** Distress from difficult experiences, but mitigated by the support of warm, responsive adults (for example, a child's loss of one parent but with the love and care of the remaining parent)

>> **Toxic:** Distress but without warm, responsive adult support (for example, abuse, neglect, or household dysfunction)

Perceiving something as stressful

Your stress-response systems enable you to respond to threats, challenges, or opportunities. Without a response, you'd be unable to manage or adapt to changing situations. You'd be like a boat adrift at sea without a sail or rudder, unable to navigate or steer through the storms and waves of life.

The Yerkes-Dodson curve

Another way to frame stress responses as neither "good" nor "bad" but adaptive is through the Yerkes-Dodson curve, shown in Figure 17-1. This inverted U shape plots stress levels against performance or the "effect" of stress, showing that not all stress is detrimental.

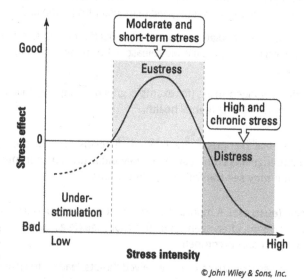

FIGURE 17-1:
The Yerkes-Dodson curve.

© John Wiley & Sons, Inc.

>> Low stress leads to boredom and poor performance.

>> Eustress motivates and promotes learning.

>> Prolonged or unmanaged stress (distress) can cause anxiety, overwhelm, and reduced performance.

Understanding the balance of stress can help you optimize your performance and manage your stress levels effectively. By recognizing your optimal stress level, you can aim to maintain it for better productivity and well-being.

Is this threat a challenge or an opportunity?

You may shift from experiencing eustress (good stress) to distress (bad stress) based more on how you perceive the stressor than on the actual challenges you face.

Cognitive Appraisal Theory helps explain this shift. When you encounter a stressor, your mind first asks, "Is this a challenge or an opportunity?" Then it evaluates, "Is this exceeding my ability to cope?" The answers to these questions vary from person to person. And they may vary for you at different ages or stages of life.

Think of it like sailing a boat. The wind represents life's challenges. When a heavy gust hits, you first decide if it's a chance to set your sail just so and speed up, or if you need to reef in your mainsail, point head to wind, and bunker down below deck. Part of that assessment is your sailing abilities and your boat's seaworthiness. If you feel prepared, you adjust your sails and enjoy the ride. If not, the same wind can feel overwhelming.

REMEMBER

We feel stressed when real or imagined pressures exceed our perceived ability to cope.

As you read this chapter on stress, you have the opportunity to think of stress using the metaphor of a sailing boat. This is a common metaphor used in psychology (and as a sailor myself, it makes a lot of sense!). Here's how I think about it:

>> Imagine yourself as the sailor navigating through the ocean of life.

>> Your crew — family, friends, teachers, colleagues, and health professionals — supports you along the way.

>> The type of boat — canoe, racing skiff, tinny, oil tanker — reflects your individual characteristics, such as age and temperament.

>> The equipment on your boat represents the resources and tools at your disposal.

>> Your learned sailing skills are your coping mechanisms and abilities to handle stress.

>> Knowledge of the sea, weather, and navigation translates to your understanding of stress and how to manage it.

>> The severity of bad weather depicts the intensity of the challenges and stressors you face.

By viewing stress this way, you can better understand and manage it, ensuring smoother sailing through both calm and stormy seas.

REMEMBER

To extend my metaphor of a sailing boat: If there's not enough wind (low stress), you're left drifting. If there's too much wind (high stress), it's difficult to control your boat and navigate effectively. However, with just the right breeze (moderate stress) and sailing skills, you can skim across the waves and enjoy the ride. This "sweet spot" of wind represents the optimal level of stress where you perform at your best, energized and in control without being overwhelmed.

Tuning into the Neuro-Symphony of Stress

There is more to your stress-response system than just the simple "fight or flight" response.

Consider the wildly different ways you are challenged: To feeling cold and hungry to feeling ostracized by your friends to hiding under a table during an earthquake to packing up your house and moving to a new city. Being able to respond to a multitude of stressors in smart, adaptable ways requires more than a "fight or flight" reaction that gets turned on or off.

An orchestrated neuro-symphony

One of my favorite academic articles, published in *Nature Reviews Neuroscience* in 2009, coined the term "neuro-symphony of stress," emphasizing how your brain coordinates a complex array of neurotransmitters, neuropeptides, and hormones to respond to stressors. These mediators act over different timeframes, from seconds to weeks, helping you adapt to both immediate and prolonged challenges.

Many factors influence how you perceive and respond to stress, which is why your brain and body need a complex repertoire. Some factors include:

>> Duration of the stressor, which can last from seconds to years (acute versus chronic)

>> Type of stressor (physical versus psychological)

>> Context (such as the time of day)

>> Your age, sex, and genetic background play a role

>> Your stages of life, from childhood to old age

Your "stress neuro-symphony" ensures that your brain and body can handle anything from a sudden scare, such as a spider jumping on you, to prolonged stress, such as caring for a dying relative. By understanding how these different mediators work together, you can better manage feeling "stressed" and experience resilience and thrive when you're challenged.

Understanding your dual stress response system

Imagine your brain and body working together in a finely tuned neuro symphony to handle the challenges, or stressors you face every day. Two major systems play leading roles:

>> Hypothalamic-Pituitary-Adrenal (HPA) axis

>> Autonomic Nervous System (ANS)

When you face an immediate stressor, such as a hairy spider or loud noise at night, your ANS kicks in with a neurally mediated quick-fire response, providing a burst of energy and alertness through the rapid release of adrenaline and neural activation of tissues such as blood vessels and your pupils.

The swift ANS response is often followed by the slower, hormone-mediated HPA axis activation, which sustains your response if the stressor persists by releasing cortisol to maintain energy supply and modulate bodily functions.

The Autonomic Nervous System: Your first responder

Your ANS plays a key role in your immediate or short-term, responses to stressors. The ANS has two main branches that work together to keep you balanced

>> Sympathetic Nervous System (SNS)

>> Parasympathetic Nervous System (PNS)

Both systems are summarized in Figure 17-2.

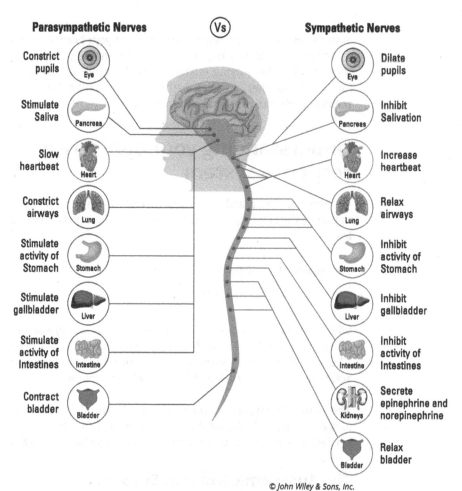

Parasympathetic Nerves (Vs) **Sympathetic Nerves**

Parasympathetic Nerves	Organ	Sympathetic Nerves
Constrict pupils	Eye	Dilate pupils
Stimulate Saliva	Pancreas	Inhibit Salivation
Slow heartbeat	Heart	Increase heartbeat
Constrict airways	Lung	Relax airways
Stimulate activity of Stomach	Stomach	Inhibit activity of Stomach
Stimulate gallbladder	Liver	Inhibit gallbladder
Stimulate activity of Intestines	Intestine	Inhibit activity of Intestines
Contract bladder	Bladder / Kidneys	Secrete epinephrine and norepinephrine
	Bladder	Relax bladder

FIGURE 17-2: Symphathetic Nervous System (SNS) and the Parasympathetic Nervous System (PNS).

© John Wiley & Sons, Inc.

SYMPATHETIC NERVOUS SYSTEM (SNS)

Think of the SNS as your body's accelerator. When you encounter a threat or challenge, the SNS triggers your body into action. This trigger is often called the "fight or flight" response. SNS activation involves:

>> Increasing heart rate and breathing rate for more blood and oxygen delivery

>> Dilates your pupils to improve your vision

>> Release of adrenaline and noradrenaline to boost energy and alertness

>> Blood vessel constriction to redirect your blood flow to essential organs and muscles

>> Inhibiting your digestion to prioritize energy for immediate action

- >> Increased glucose release to provide you immediate energy
- >> Sweat production to keep you cool

PARASYMPATHETIC NERVOUS SYSTEM (PSNS)

The PSNS is like your body's brake system. After an immediate threat has passed, the PSNS helps you calm down. Sometimes this is called the "rest and digest" state. PSNS activation involves:

- >> Slowing your heart rate and breathing to conserve energy
- >> Stimulating relaxation to help you recover and restore balance
- >> Constricting your pupil size for close-up vision
- >> Increasing blood flow to your gut to enhance nutrient absorption and digestion
- >> Resuming urination and bowel movements

WARNING

Looking at that list, it's worth pointing out that not every action of the PNS is about recovering from scary events! Together with the SNS, the PNS plays a vital role in maintaining regular physiological function and ensuring overall homeostasis.

The HPA axis: Your extended defense

Your HPA axis consists of three components — hypothalamus, pituitary gland, and adrenal glands — that work together to help you respond to stressors over a longer timeframe than the ANS.

Here's a quick breakdown of its key components:

- >> **Hypothalamus:** Acts as the command center, releasing corticotropin-releasing hormone (CRH) when a stressor is perceived.
- >> **Pituitary Gland:** Releases adrenocorticotropic hormone (ACTH) into your bloodstream in response to CRH.
- >> **Adrenal Glands:** Release cortisol, the "stress hormone," when triggered by ACTH. Sit on top of the kidneys.

Cortisol plays a crucial role in helping you manage stress by triggering a range of immediate actions throughout your body and brain. (See "Understanding Stress Hormones" in the following section.) When cortisol levels rise, it signals to the hypothalamus and pituitary to reduce the release of CRH and ACTH, respectively. This feedback loop helps cortisol self-regulate its own release, preventing excessive levels that can be harmful.

Understanding stress hormones

Adrenaline, noradrenaline, and cortisol are three key signaling molecules that orchestrate your brain and body's response to threats, challenges, and opportunities.

Release and roles of adrenaline and noradrenaline

REMEMBER

Adrenaline and noradrenaline are known in the U.S. as epinephrine and norepinephrine.

Here's what you need to know:

>> **Noradrenaline** acts both as a hormone (increasing heart rate, blood flow, and regulating blood vessel constriction) and as a neurotransmitter in the brain (increasing arousal, alertness, vigilance, and memory formation). It's produced by neurons in the locus coeruleus in the brainstem.

>> **Adrenaline** (released by the adrenal medulla) quickly increases heart rate, breathing, dilates pupils, and releases glucose.

Release and roles of cortisol

When you encounter a threat or challenge, your body releases cortisol from your adrenal glands, located atop your kidneys. Cortisol has several actions designed to help you respond and adapt to stressors by:

>> Promoting glucose release for quick energy

>> Regulating metabolism of fats, proteins, and carbs

>> Enhancing alertness, focus, and memory

Cortisol acts by binding to two types of receptors: the glucocorticoid receptor and the mineralocorticoid receptor. The effects of cortisol depend largely on the number and location of these receptors. The receptors respond differently based on cortisol levels over time:

>> **Chronic high levels:** Can lead to a decrease in the number of receptors (downregulation), making tissues less sensitive to cortisol.

>> **Prolonged low levels:** Can increase the number of receptors (upregulation), making tissues more sensitive to cortisol.

WARNING

Problems can start to emerge when cortisol or adrenaline release continues for extended periods. This can lead to receptor desensitization and dysregulation, contributing to various health issues such as chronic inflammation, anxiety, depression, and metabolic disorders.

It's worth noting that cortisol also follows a diurnal (daily) pattern, with levels peaking in the early morning to help wake you up and gradually declining throughout the day. This daily rhythm helps regulate your sleep-wake cycle, energy levels, and overall daily rhythm.

REMEMBER

Adrenaline, noradrenaline, and cortisol are key hormones in your body's stress response. Their release is "tonically active," meaning they are not simply switched on or off in response to threats. Instead, their levels adjust like a volume dial, turning up or down as needed, like instruments in an orchestra where each hormone plays its part.

Decoding fight, flight, freeze, and fawn

The concepts of fight, flight, freeze, and fawn (sometimes called befriend) are useful metaphors to describe how humans and other animals respond to threats. But it's very important to realize these responses vary greatly depending on the individual and the specific threat. For instance, deer and gazelles are both herding animals preyed upon by predators, but their strategies differ significantly. For example,

>> Deer freeze and rely more on camouflage to avoid detection, blending into their surroundings to stay safe.

>> Gazelles flee depend on their speed and agility to escape predators in the open savannas, often outrunning them with quick, agile movements.

>> Lions fight fiercely to defend their territory from an intruder, displaying a more aggressive and territorial response.

>> When an elephant calf is threatened, the entire herd circles around it to protect it from predators, showcasing a strong fawning response.

Humans react with a mix of all types of responses and what happens when depends on multiple interacting factors and contexts.

FREEZE RESPONSE

The freeze response, often the initial reaction to a threat, lets you "stop, look, and listen." This hypervigilant state helps you assess the situation. By remaining still, prey can avoid detection by predators that primarily see movement. This response is associated with heightened alertness and caution.

FLIGHT AND FIGHT RESPONSES

Following the freeze response, you may be lucky enough to flee from danger. If an escape route isn't possible, all that's left for you to do is fight. But this sequence — flight then fight — doesn't always play out. For example, someone trained in martial arts, or a large, strong male may be more likely to fight an attacker in a dark car park, while a young teenage girl may try to flee.

BEFRIEND RESPONSE

The "tend and befriend" or "fawn" response is the idea that humans often seek social support when we're stressed. When you face a threat, you may tend to your children for their protection or call your Mum or Dad for mutual support and comfort (my default is always to call my Mum on the phone). This response is driven by neurocircuitry involving oxytocin and endogenous opioid peptides. These chemicals encourage bonding and can help reduce your stress, providing a calming effect, and promoting social cohesion.

TIP

Like all behaviors, your reactions depend on your experiences and culture. In Australia, many people welcome our enormous but harmless, mosquito-catching huntsman spiders into their homes. But if you're visiting for the first time, you might freeze in terror and reach for bug spray (or even the vacuum!).

Stress hormones and immune health

Think about times when you burned the candle at both ends. Perhaps you had to work late, juggling family caregiving or barely finding a moment to catch your breath. Then, just when you finally got a weekend to relax, boom — you caught a cold. This familiar connection between stress and immune function is something scientists have been exploring for years, and the more they learn, the more it confirms what you intuitively know — that stress messes with your health.

Your immune system has two main arms:

>> Innate immune response, which provides immediate, non-specific defense against pathogens.

>> Adaptive immune response, which is slower but more specific, targeting pathogens and creating memory cells for faster future responses.

Acute stress boosts immunity, but chronic stress has the opposite effect. Psychological or physical stressors (like deadlines, grief, or injuries) trigger stress hormones like cortisol. Prolonged stress can suppress the immune system, reducing lymphocytes (white blood cells), which makes you more prone to illness.

But this isn't a one-way conversation! Your immune system can also impact your brain and even mood. For example, during infection, cytokines (immune-signaling molecules) can lead to fatigue, depression, or anxiety. Inflammation can even alter social behavior, causing "sickness behaviors" where you want to curl up at home alone, hidden from others.

REMEMBER

When you're sick, your body becomes more vulnerable, making you more alert to social threats and encouraging you to seek solace at home. This two-way relationship means that not only do threats or challenges affect your immune system, but your immune responses can also influence how you feel and behave.

Mapping the Impact of Stress on Brain Terrain

Everyone responds to stress differently. Remember, Australians may befriend hairy huntsman spiders, whereas visitors may see them as deadly threats. This reminds us that stress responses aren't inherently good or bad; they vary widely and depend on context. It's prolonged or excessive stress that leads to wear and tear on the body and brain.

Viewing the brain as a stress organ

The brain plays a crucial role in how you respond to stress. The late neuroscience Professor Bruce McEwan, who first discovered toxic stress has a profound effect on the brain, outlines three main reasons why the brain is involved:

>> **Interpreting stress:** Your brain identifies threats and decides what is stressful.

>> **Regulating your responses:** It controls behavioral and physiological reactions to stress through various systems, affecting adaptation or health.

>> **Target of stress:** Stress changes the brain's structure and function, influencing gene expression and embedding experiences.

McEwan's research, initially on the hippocampus, now includes areas like the amygdala and prefrontal cortex, related to memory and self-regulation. These changes can be reversed through exercise, therapy, social support, good sleep, and a balanced diet.

Brain regions most vulnerable to stress

Your brain is directly affected by stress and stress-related hormones, especially cortisol. Under normal conditions, these stress hormones help your brain adapt and respond. But when stress is excessive, chronic, or toxic, it can cause damage. Stress impacts not only the hippocampus, which is involved in memory, but also other brain regions like the amygdala and prefrontal cortex (PFC), which are involved in fear, working memory, and self-control.

Allostasis and allostatic load

Allostasis is your body's and brain's ability to maintain stability through change. To stay healthy, your body continuously adjusts its internal systems to respond to external demands. However, when stressors are toxic or chronic, your body's ability to cope is overwhelmed, leading to allostatic overload.

These concepts help us understand that stress responses can be both protective and damaging, affecting your brain and body in complex ways. Understanding allostasis and allostatic load has been crucial for integrating the biology of stress with psychosocial factors, helping fields like health psychology, medicine, and psychiatry better address stress-related disorders.

Wear and tear on your brain and body

Allostatic load includes the cumulative impact of life events (that may be stressors), and the physiological consequences of health-damaging behaviors such as poor sleep, lack of exercise, smoking, excessive alcohol consumption, and an unhealthy diet. When these various challenges exceed your ability to cope, allostatic overload occurs.

REMEMBER

In summary, allostatic load is how much stress your body and brain are under. It shows just how important it is to both manage your response to stressors and the importance of healthy lifestyle habits to lessen the negative effects of long-term stress.

Navigating life stages and stress vulnerability

Certain stages of life make you more vulnerable to the impacts of stress. These are typically ages or life stages when the brain is undergoing rapid change such as critical periods of development or later-in-life aging. You may like to look at Chapters 6 through 8 for more information about brain health through the lifespan.

- » **Infancy and childhood:** The brain's plasticity during this time allows for rapid learning but also makes it vulnerable to lasting effects from toxic stress, such as abuse or neglect, which can impact long-term health.

- » **Adolescence:** Teens experience rapid brain development and are especially sensitive to stress. Providing a supportive environment while managing your own stress helps teens build resilience without being overwhelmed by toxic stress.

- » **Pregnancy and motherhood:** The brain reorganizes during pregnancy, but severe stress can disrupt this, increasing risks for anxiety and affecting the baby's health. Strong social support is key to buffering against these effects.

- » **Aging:** As you age, your brain becomes more susceptible to stress, with higher cortisol levels and reduced brain volume. Prolonged stress can accelerate cognitive decline and memory issues, with recovery mechanisms less effective over time.

Recognizing the health risks of toxic or chronic stress

As a reminder, stress — like sleep, diet, exercise, genes, relationships — is just one risk factor for disease.

Experiencing prolonged or excessive stress often adds considerable weight tipping the healthy balance toward a greater allostatic load, disease, and dysfunction. Throughout this book you consider many different health issues — ranging from cardiovascular diseases to mental health disorders to dementia. It won't come as a surprise to you that all are exacerbated by chronic or toxic stress. Here's a list of well-established health consequences of toxic or chronic stress.

POST-TRAUMATIC STRESS DISORDER (PTSD)

Post-Traumatic Stress Disorder (PTSD) is a complex mental health condition that can develop after experiencing or witnessing trauma. It affects 7 to 8 percent of people in the United States, with higher rates among veterans, emergency workers, and women. Symptoms include flashbacks, nightmares, extreme anxiety, and intrusive thoughts.

PTSD involves heightened activity in the amygdala (fear processing) and reduced regulation by the prefrontal cortex. The sympathetic nervous system is often over-activated, triggering intense fight-or-flight responses even without immediate danger.

(continued)

(continued)

Treatment usually combines psychotherapy, trauma-focused CBT, and medications like SSRIs. Australia recently approved psychedelic treatments for PTSD, available only through psychiatrists in controlled settings. Eye Movement Desensitization and Reprocessing (EMDR) therapy has also shown significant success, despite its unclear neurobiology. Early intervention and a supportive environment are crucial for recovery, helping individuals regain control and move forward.

>> **Burnout:** a state of exhaustion caused by long-term stress, often related to work or caregiving, leaving you feeling drained and unmotivated.

>> **Anxiety:** Chronic stress keeps your body and brain on high alert, leading to constant worry and tension, which can develop into anxiety disorders.

>> **Depression:** Chronic stress can lead to biochemical changes in the brain, causing mood regulation issues and potentially leading to depression.

>> **Poor cardiovascular health:** Chronic stress produces cortisol and adrenaline, which can damage your heart and blood vessels over time, increasing the risk of heart disease.

>> **Metabolic issues:** Stress can alter your metabolism, leading to weight gain and raising the risk of diabetes and other metabolic problems. I discuss metabolic syndrome in Chapter 19.

>> **Weakened immune system:** Chronic stress weakens your immune system, making you more prone to infections and illnesses.

>> **Sleep problems:** Stress often disrupts sleep, leading to a vicious cycle that worsens brain, body, and mental health.

Cultivating Resilience and Growth

Your ANS and HPA axis help you adapt to challenges, but prolonged exposure to stress hormones like cortisol can take a toll on your health, increasing risks for immune, metabolic, heart, and mental health issues, and even speeding up aging. The key is learning to manage stress and build resilience, which helps you recover, adapt to adversity, and maintain well-being.

Theories of resilience

Resilience has plenty of definitions, both in pop culture and academia. Here are a few different ways of defining resilience that I quite like:

>> **Resilience is like sailing a boat.** It's not about avoiding rough seas but knowing how to adjust your sails and steer your course, using your skills and the support of your crew to weather the storm and keep moving forward (as a sailor, this is obviously my favorite!).

>> **Resilience is like bamboo: Flexible yet strong.** Resilience is the ability to bend with challenges and bounce back without breaking, like flexible yet strong bamboo.

>> **Resilience** is the process of adapting well in the face of adversity, trauma, tragedy, threats, or significant sources of stress (according to the American Psychological Association).

>> **Resilience is influenced by multiple environmental systems,** from immediate family and friends to broader societal and cultural contexts according to the Ecological Systems Theory proposed by Urie Bronfenbrenner.

Resilience: trait, state, or process?

You may think about resilience as something you're born with — you're either resilient or not — or maybe you see resilience as a skill you've learned over time. Academics like to muse over these sorts of ideas too and one of the most common discussions is whether resilience is a trait, a state, or a process.

>> **Trait resilience** means some people naturally have qualities such as optimism and mental toughness that help them handle stress better.

>> **State resilience** suggests your ability to cope can change depending on the situation — sometimes you feel like you're coping well, other times you're falling in a weeping heap.

>> **Process resilience** is about how you can grow and become more resilient over time through various life experiences.

REMEMBER

Understanding these different angles can help you see that resilience isn't just something you either have or don't have. You can develop and improve resilience, no matter your starting point.

Building protective relationships

Building resilience isn't just about you being stoic or as my dad used to say feeling "10-foot tall and bullet-proof." Resilience is also about the people around you who support you and your ability to cope with whatever life throws your way. Despite their different academic approaches, many resilience theories emphasize other people as importance in building and sustaining resilience.

For more detailed insights on how social relationships protect mental health and brain aging, refer to Chapters 8 and 15. These chapters delve deeper into the role of supportive networks and social interactions in fostering resilience and maintaining mental well-being throughout life.

Embracing calm with mindfulness and meditation

Mindfulness and meditation have roots in ancient practices. But in the last couple of decades, scientific interest has grown in exploring their benefits for mental and physical health.

The two words mindfulness and meditation often go hand in hand, but more formally are defined as follows:

>> **Mindfulness** is being aware of your thoughts, feelings, and surroundings moment by moment without judgment, often cultivated through meditation or daily activities.

>> **Meditation** is set of practices to train attention and awareness, aiming for a clear, calm, and stable mental state, with various forms like mindfulness or mantra-based meditation.

Mindfulness-Based Stress Reduction (MBSR)

One of the most well-known and researched mindfulness programs is Mindfulness-Based Stress Reduction (MBSR), which was developed by Jon Kabat-Zinn, professor of medicine and student of Zen Buddhist monks. MBSR combines mindfulness meditation with body awareness and yoga to help reduce stress and improve overall well-being. It's been taught the world over and has been the subject of various trials and even metanalyses of its effectiveness.

Here are some specific benefits participants report:

>> **Mental benefits:** Participants report more energy, enthusiasm, improved focus, and concentration, making it easier to stay present and on task.

>> **Emotional and mental health benefits:** MBSR increases resilience to stress and fosters greater compassion for others, making it more actionable. It helps reduce anxiety and depression symptoms (though not better than other treatments).

>> **Physical and mental health improvements:** Modest improvements in physical health, like better sleep and pain management.

TIP

There are nearly unlimited options for you to learn MBSR, both online and in-person. Many towns and cities have mindfulness centers that offer MBSR courses. You can also consider local health centers, yoga studies, or even ask your family doctor. A quick internet search with your location can help you find nearby options!

WARNING

While mindfulness and meditation are often touted as cure-alls for stress and mental health issues, it's crucial to approach them with a balanced perspective. These practices are rooted in ancient wisdom and backed by modern neuroscience, but they are not the definitive solution for everyone.

Breathing through breathwork

I know this sounds like taking something as basic as breathing and turning it into "work." But before you roll your eyes, hear me out. There is some evidence that focusing on your breath can be a simple yet powerful way to reduce stress and improve overall well-being. But, like all techniques, you may need to practice.

There are numerous positive health outcomes measured in people practicing deep breathing. These beneficial outcomes include:

>> **Cardiovascular benefits:** Increased heart rate variability, reduced heart rate, and lower blood pressure

>> **Respiratory benefits:** Increased tissue oxygenation, decreased carbon dioxide levels, and better lung capacity and function

>> **Stress and mental health benefits:** Activation of the parasympathetic nervous system, reduced cortisol, enhanced mental focus, and improved emotional regulation

Here are a few of the more well-known ways of doing "breath work") to reduce stress:

>> **Physiological sigh:** Inhale deeply through the nose, followed by a second shorter inhale, then slowly exhale through your mouth (as if through a straw).

>> **Box breathing:** Inhale for four counts, hold for four, exhale for four, and pause for four before repeating. Navy SEALs use it to stay calm and focused.

>> **4-7-8 breathing:** Inhale for four seconds, hold for seven, and exhale for eight. A variation on box breathing with a different rhythm.

>> **Diaphragmatic breathing:** Breathe deeply into the diaphragm, not the chest, feeling your belly rise while keeping your chest still.

Prescribing Calm

You've probably heard it a million times: "Mindfulness is the key to managing stress." While this sentiment is well-intentioned, it can sometimes feel like trying to fit a square peg into a round hole (and it doesn't always work that well for this author either!).

Here is a list of different strategies you can mix and match to create your toolkit for navigating life's inevitable gusts and gales.

Mind-body practices (physiological regulation):

>> Practice deep breathing exercises such as box breathing, diaphragmatic breathing, or the 4-7-8 technique.

>> Mindfulness meditation practices, for example MBSR.

>> Cold water swimming or ice baths release endorphins improving your mood.

>> Regular exercise, which includes everything from walking to team sports to gym sessions.

>> Relaxation techniques such as progressive muscle relaxation, visualization, or guided imagery to reduce physical tension.

>> Activities such as tai chi or qigong combine gentle physical movements with mindfulness.

Preventatives (lifestyle and habits):

>> Maintain a balanced diet of fruits, vegetables, lean proteins, and whole grains.

>> Ensure you get regular quality sleep every night.

>> Limit caffeine and alcohol.

>> Take regular breaks from screens and social media.

>> Keep a gratitude journal to focus on positive aspects of your life.

>> Learn to say no and set personal and professional boundaries to protect your time and reduce your risk of burnout.

>> Prioritizing tasks, set realistic goals, and take breaks to manage your workload effectively.

Social interventions (support and community):

>> Build and maintain strong relationships with friends and family.

>> Seek out therapy or counseling.

>> Engage with your community by volunteering to create a sense of purpose and connection.

Additional approaches (hobbies and personal interests):

>> Indulge in those activities or hobbies you enjoy, such as reading, gardening, painting, or playing music, to relax and unwind.

>> Spend time outdoors in green or blue spaces.

>> Write your thoughts and feelings down in a journal to process emotions and gain perspective.

>> Laugh! Watch a funny movie, read a good book, or spend time with people who make you laugh.

>> Use art, music, dance, or writing to relieve emotions and stress.

TIP

To conclude, just as I've taught my boys, both young sailors and salty old seadogs know that calm seas, gentle breezes, howling southerlies, the odd shark sighting, and big swells are all part of the adventure. What's important is understanding and managing their boat and knowing when to tack and gybe, go head to wind, when to call into a safe port, and when to call the coastguard!

By equipping yourself with various stress management techniques — whether they involve strengthening your mind-body connection, adopting preventative lifestyle habits, seeking social support, or engaging in hobbies — you can maintain your boat's seaworthiness. Remember, it's not about avoiding the storms, but rather learning how to adjust your sails to harness its power, ensuring you can steer your course.

Chapter **18**

Rethinking Drugs and Alcohol

Picture this: You're at a lively party, and conversations and laughter are flowing as freely as the drinks. But have you ever paused to wonder what's happening inside your brain as you sip your glass of Shiraz? And (depending on where in the world you live or who you party with) maybe there's a cannabis gummy or a line of cocaine on offer. Have you considered how that relaxed state or euphoric high may impact your brain in the long run?

From the immediate euphoria to potential long-term consequences, this chapter takes a brief look at how these substances (some legal, others illicit) interact with your brain. I explore the sobering reality of alcohol use disorder, the therapeutic promises and risks of marijuana and psychedelics, and the emerging trend of micro-dosing pharmaceuticals for cognitive enhancement.

WARNING

The research is rapidly evolving, so keep in mind that this chapter aims to provide you with a look at the brain health effects only. I want to acknowledge that laws surrounding these substances vary significantly across different parts of the world, and that moral and ethical perspectives on their use are deeply personal and culturally influenced. My focus here is purely on the basics of brain health, without stepping out of our lane into the complex territories of legality, morality, or ethics.

Assessing Alcohol's Effect on Brain Health

Alcohol has been a part of human culture for millennia, dating back to biblical times, and is part of many religious traditions and daily diets. Beyond the initial buzz, drinking can lead to a range of adverse outcomes. In the short term, being drunk increases your risk of accidents, injuries, and impaired judgment. Longer-term, habitual drinking can lead to chronic health issues such as liver disease, heart problems, and mental health disorders.

Long-term consequences for brain health

Risky drinking leads to changes in brain structure and network connectivity. Studies show that heavy drinking (three or more drinks a day for women and four or more for men) causes widespread brain changes, especially in areas such as the frontal cortex, hippocampus, and cerebellum.

People with Alcohol Use Disorder (AUD) show lower grey matter volume in key regions such as the prefrontal cortex, insula, and thalamus, with damage linked to the amount and duration of alcohol consumption. Alcohol also leads to white matter degeneration in structures like the corpus callosum, affecting the brain's ability to process information. These brain changes can worsen with age, emphasizing the long-term impact of chronic alcohol use on brain health.

Drinking alcohol at risky levels can lead to alcohol-related brain injury (ARBI), which affects your thinking, memory, personality, and movement. Two well-known types of ARBI are:

>> **Wernicke's Encephalopathy:** Sudden brain swelling due to severe thiamine deficiency, causing eye movement issues, poor coordination, and confusion.

>> **Korsakoff's Syndrome:** Chronic memory problems and difficulty learning new information.

While anyone can develop ARBI, it's most common in men over 45 with a long history of heavy drinking. The good news is that some of the damage can be reversed if you stop drinking and get treatment early.

Alcohol Use Disorder

Alcohol Use Disorder (AUD) is a medical condition where you find it hard to stop or control your drinking, even when it's causing problems in your life.

TIP

AUD is the term that's used nowadays to include what people commonly refer to as alcohol abuse, dependence, addiction, or alcoholism. AUD can range from mild to severe and affects the brain, making it easier to relapse.

Who's at risk for AUD?

Your risk for AUD increases with how much and how often you drink. Starting to drink at a young age, having a family history of alcohol problems, and experiencing mental health issues or trauma can all raise your chances of developing AUD. In short, AUD risk is influenced by a combination of biological, psychological, and social factors.

If you answer "yes" to questions such as these, you may have AUD:

» Do you drink more or longer than you intended?

» Have you tried to cut down but couldn't?

» Does drinking interfere with your daily responsibilities?

» Do you continue to drink despite problems with family or friends?

» Do you experience withdrawal symptoms when not drinking?

The more symptoms you have, the more urgent it is to seek help.

Getting treatment for AUD

You have several ways to treat AUD, and what works for one person may not work for another. Options include:

» **Medications:** Naltrexone, acamprosate, and disulfiram can help reduce cravings and prevent relapse.

» **Behavioral Treatments:** Therapy sessions that focus on changing drinking behaviors and developing coping skills.

» **Support Groups:** Peer support from groups such as Alcoholics Anonymous can be very helpful, especially when combined with other treatments.

REMEMBER

Recovery is possible, but it often requires ongoing effort and professional support. Early treatment can help you develop skills to avoid triggers and manage stress, making it easier to maintain sobriety. If you or someone you know is struggling with alcohol use, don't hesitate to seek help.

EVEN MODERATE DRINKING AFFECTS THE BRAIN

A 2022 study using data from 36,678 participants in the UK Biobank found that even light to moderate drinking is linked to negative changes in brain structure, including reduced brain volume and poorer white matter integrity. These effects are noticeable in people consuming just one to two units of alcohol daily and worsen with higher intake, highlighting the potential harm of moderate drinking on brain health.

TIP

A good search to use for someone seeking help for their drinking is **alcohol addiction help near me** or **alcohol support services in [your location]**.

Assessing potential positive effects of alcohol

In Chapter 12, we looked at the Blue Zones, regions where people live significantly longer and healthier lives. One habit for many people in these areas is the tradition of "Wine at 5." Some scientists argue that the occasional glass of wine shared with friends or family can actually have some health benefits.

While the debate over the health benefits and risks of red wine continues, those who champion its virtues do so for one main reason: Polyphenols such as resveratrol — naturally occurring compounds in the skins of red grapes that have antioxidant properties. These antioxidants fight off oxidative stress and inflammation.

The evidence on alcohol's health impact is far from perfect (as is all research on diet and nutrition). But here's a good news story to balance out all the discussions of risky drinking and AUD. A 2024 study using data from the UK Biobank, from over 500,000 participants, explored how different types of alcoholic drinks affect risks of death, heart disease, and kidney disease. At the start of the study, participants shared details about their drinking habits, including what they drank (for example, champagne, white or red wine, beer, and spirits) and how often. Over about 12 years of follow up, 2,852 participants reported kidney disease, 79,958 reported heart disease, and 18,923 participants died.

The study found that total alcohol consumption showed a U-shaped curve for heart disease and death, meaning moderate drinkers had lower risks compared to heavy drinkers and non-drinkers (which includes past drinkers).

"Safe" drinking limits were identified. These align pretty closely with the Australian guidelines, especially concerning weekly consumption limits.

>> Total alcohol: <11 grams/day for men, <10 grams/day for women

>> Red wine: <7 glasses/week for men, <6 glasses/week for women

>> Champagne plus white wine: <5 glasses/week

>> Fortified wine: <4 glasses/week

The results of the study tend to suggest you can get away with a few glasses *of wine* per week, but it's essential to drink responsibly.

REMEMBER

In summary, while there is some evidence that moderate alcohol consumption may have health benefits, it is important to consider the potential risks and to drink responsibly. Always consult with a healthcare provider to determine what is best for your individual health.

Understanding Cannabis' Influence on the Brain

Cannabis has a long history of use for both its mind-altering and medicinal properties. Its popularity surged in the 1960s, when it became known by various names you may have heard of such as hemp, hashish, bud, ganja, reefer, weed, pot, grass, dope, and Mary Jane. While cannabis has potential therapeutic benefits, such as pain relief and reduced anxiety, it also carries risks. Any drug capable of producing a beneficial effect also carries the potential for negative side effects.

Getting up to speed on the basics of cannabis

Before we dive into the details of what cannabis is and how it works, I should remind you that cannabis laws vary depending on where you live. In many countries, it's illegal with strict penalties. In some places, it's decriminalized, meaning you can use it without facing criminal charges. Other regions allow cannabis strictly for medical use with a prescription. And then there are places where it's fully legal for both medical and recreational use. These laws reflect different cultural attitudes, public health policies, and political climates.

What is cannabis?

When you use cannabis, it acts as a CNS depressant, slowing down your brain activity and making you feel chilled out, relaxed, happy, and sociable. You usually feel the effects immediately after smoking or vaping it, but they can also last for several hours after use. You also may find yourself laughing more, experiencing heightened senses, or feeling very hungry.

Cannabis, also known as marijuana, is a plant that contains many different chemical compounds known as cannabinoids, including tetrahydrocannabinol (THC) and cannabidiol (CBD).

>> THC is the primary psychoactive compound in cannabis, responsible for the high that users experience.

>> CBD is non-psychoactive and is often used for its potential therapeutic benefits, such as reducing anxiety, inflammation, and pain.

Many people use cannabis recreationally for its mind-altering effects — tapping into the THC. The experience can vary from relaxation and euphoria to altered sensory perception and time distortion. Medicinal cannabis is used in the treatment of various medical conditions, including chronic pain, epilepsy, multiple sclerosis, and to help people undergoing chemotherapy to prevent nausea and vomiting. CBD has been studied for its potential health benefits without the intoxicating effects of THC.

REMEMBER

How you consume cannabis matters: Smoking it gives you a quick, short high, while eating it as an edible means a slower onset and a longer-lasting effect. Regular users develop some tolerance, but it's not as intense as with drugs such as cocaine or alcohol.

How does cannabis work?

THC and CBD interact with the endocannabinoid system in your body, which plays a key role in regulating various physiological processes.

Endocannabinoids are naturally occurring molecules similar to the cannabinoids found in cannabis. Endocannabinoids and cannabinoids all bind to the two main cannabinoid receptors:

>> **CB1 receptors:** Found in the brain and central nervous system, they influence coordination, movement, pain, appetite, memory, and mood.

>> **CB2 receptors:** Found mostly in the immune system and peripheral tissues, they modulate inflammation and immune response.

THC binds primarily to CB1 receptors. This interaction is responsible for THC's psychoactive effects, such as euphoria, altered perception, and relaxation.

CBD, on the other hand, does not bind strongly to CB1 or CB2 receptors. CB2 receptors are mainly located in the immune system and peripheral tissues. Instead, CBD influences the endocannabinoid system indirectly by enhancing the levels of endocannabinoids in your system and interacting with other receptors. This can help reduce inflammation, pain, and anxiety without causing a high.

The benefits of cannabis

REMEMBER

Medicinal cannabis is primarily used for therapeutic purposes, distinct from its recreational counterpart, which is often consumed for its mind-altering effects. Medicinal cannabis products usually contain THC, CBD, or a combination of both. They're synthesized in laboratories to mimic the effects of naturally occurring chemicals in cannabis and usually taken orally (not smoked).

In Australia, medicinal cannabis is prescribed for various conditions, including arthritis pain, lower back pain, neck pain, neuropathic pain, anxiety, cancer-related symptoms like pain and nausea, epilepsy, insomnia, and multiple sclerosis (MS).

Other health benefits of medicinal cannabis include increased appetite and reduced nausea, especially for cancer patients undergoing chemotherapy, lowered eye pressure for glaucoma patients, reduced anxiety, and improved sleep quality, particularly for those with PTSD, as cannabis can reduce REM sleep and nightmares.

The health risks of cannabis

You may know people who use cannabis for fun or for the same reasons others use it medically such as for pain relief or to reduce anxiety.

REMEMBER

But here's the catch: Recreational use is often unregulated and illegal in many places. This means higher risks for you when it comes to dosage, quality, and even legal trouble. In some parts of the world, you can walk into a shop and buy cannabis gummies. In other parts of the world, just having cannabis in your pocket could land you in jail.

This stark difference fuels a lot of debates about whether cannabis is beneficial or risky. Supporters tell you that cannabis offers significant therapeutic benefits and should be accessible to everyone. On the flip side, opponents worry about potential health risks and the broader impact on society.

Acknowledging the side effects

Just like any drug, cannabis comes with positive effects and negative side effects.

>> **Short-term side effects of medicinal cannabis:** Fatigue, dizziness, nausea, fever, appetite changes, dry mouth, and diarrhea.

>> **High-THC side effects:** Feeling high, sadness, hallucinations, paranoia, delusions, or difficulty distinguishing reality.

>> **Long-term effects (usually in heavy recreational users):** Cognitive decline in attention, processing speed, and memory; potential IQ drop (especially with early use); and poorer sleep quality over time.

Exploring the psychiatric risks of cannabis use in teens

The risk to mental health is one of the major concerns when it comes to discussion around the use or legalization of cannabis. Not everyone agrees that the association between cannabis use and the earlier age at onset of psychosis is causal meaning using directly causes psychosis. Some people argue that other factors, such as your genes may play a more significant role. Despite these differing opinions, it's crucial to examine the evidence and understand the potential risks, especially for teenagers and young adults.

In 2011, a significant meta-analysis of 83 studies was published by Australian researchers in *JAMA Psychiatry*. It examined the impact of cannabis on the age of onset of psychosis, including schizophrenia, in users compared to non-users. This extensive analysis involved data from over 8,000 cannabis users and more than 14,000 non-users, providing a robust dataset for conclusions.

The study found that individuals who used cannabis experienced the onset of psychotic disorders approximately 2.7 years earlier than non-users. This suggests a strong link between cannabis use and an earlier onset of psychosis, which is a significant concern. The association was particularly pronounced among younger teenagers and in studies with higher proportions of cannabis users. Additionally, the effect was more significant among males.

WARNING

In short, this study shows that cannabis may act as a trigger for psychosis, especially in those who are genetically predisposed. If you're a teenager or a young adult, waiting until adulthood before considering cannabis use is the smartest move.

Probing the Use of Psychedelics

After decades of prohibition and stigmatization, psychedelics have emerged as a promising treatment for those with mental health conditions.

What are psychedelics?

Psychedelics are a group of powerful psychoactive substances that alter perception, mood, and various cognitive processes. The term "psychedelic" comes from the Greek words *psyche*, meaning mind, and *delein*, meaning manifest.

Essentially, these substances can bring about significant changes in your mental state and perception of reality. The most well-known psychedelics include:

>> **Psilocybin:** Found in certain types of mushrooms, often referred to as "magic mushrooms"

>> **MDMA:** Commonly known as ecstasy, it's popular in party scenes but has therapeutic uses

>> **LSD:** A synthetic substance known for its potent effects on the mind

>> **DMT:** The active ingredient in the traditional South American brew ayahuasca

How do psychedelics affect the brain?

When you take a psychedelic, it specifically targets and activates serotonin (5HT) receptors in your brain, leading to altered states of consciousness and perception. This is quite different from typical antidepressants, which generally increase serotonin levels by stopping its removal from the synaptic cleft.

Psychedelics work by activating a particular subtype of serotonin receptors (5-HT2A) on neurons. These receptors are densely concentrated in areas of the brain crucial for cognitive processing, behavior control, and memory, particularly in the frontal cortex. This reception activation doesn't just cause "tripping," it also triggers multiple signaling pathways within neurons, leading to long-lasting changes in brain structure and function — the process you know as neuroplasticity.

Therapeutic use of psychedelics

Psychedelics are still illegal in many parts of the world, and their possession or use can result in legal consequences including jail time.

REMEMBER

However, in 2023, Australia made headlines by becoming the first country to approve the medicinal use of MDMA and psilocybin for certain mental health conditions. This move reflects recognition and advocacy from some groups pointing towards the potential benefits of psychedelics when used in a controlled, therapeutic setting.

Clinical trials have shown that substances such as psilocybin can rapidly relieve symptoms of depression, with effects that can last for at least a year. Psilocybin has also shown promise in treating alcohol use disorder, nicotine addiction, and end-of-life anxiety in terminally ill patients.

WARNING

In a clinical setting, psychedelics are administered under the watchful eye of trained professionals who can steer your experience safely and ensure you don't end up hugging a tree for dear life.

Micro-dosing with psychedelics

Micro-dosing is a newer trend you may associate with students cramming for finals or "tech bros" trying to hack their brains for maximum productivity. Micro-dosing involves taking very small doses of psychedelic drugs, such as LSD or psilocybin. These doses are so tiny that they don't cause the typical hallucinogenic effects but users say enhances their cognitive functions, creativity, and even mood.

The idea is that these tiny doses subtly tweak your brain's chemistry. For example, LSD and psilocybin work by interacting with serotonin receptors, which are crucial for mood regulation and cognition. By activating these receptors, even in small amounts, its said you can boost creativity, improve focus, and come up with groundbreaking ideas — all without the full-blown psychedelic trip.

WARNING

While micro-dosing may sound like the ultimate brain hack for students and tech bros alike, it's essential to weigh the potential benefits against the risks and legal implications.

Prescribing Healthy Imbibing

Let's be real: Lots of us have our vices. Whether it's a glass of wine after a long day, a hit from a vape, or exploring therapeutic effects of illicit substances, everyone has something they turn to for comfort or stress relief. The key is understanding how these substances affect your brain and overall health and then being smart about what do with that info.

Different substances have different effects. While some may help with relaxation and social bonding, others may impair your judgment and motor skills. It's important to weigh the immediate benefits against potential long-term risks. For instance, while a cannabis gummy may help with anxiety, heavy use can lead to cognitive impairments over time.

REMEMBER

Your brain is a remarkable organ, capable of incredible feats. By understanding how substances such as alcohol, cannabis, and psychedelics affect it, you can make choices that support its health and longevity. Remember, it's not about perfection but balance. So, cheers to making smart, informed decisions for a healthier brain and a happier life!

IN THIS CHAPTER

» **Understanding metabolism**

» **Avoiding metabolic syndrome**

» **Knowing how metabolism and brain health link**

» **Protecting your heart to protect your brain**

» **Making healthy lifestyle choices**

Chapter **19**

Avoiding Metabolic Syndrome

I magine your brain and body having a catch-up conversation over coffee: "Brain, why are you acting so vague today?" the body asks. "Well, Body," says the brain, "Your blood sugar is unstable, your blood pressure is way too high, and I know this is not going to make me popular, but you've put on more weight than is healthy, and all that's affecting my mood and focus!" This conversation is a bit silly (I'm sorry for the cringe) but it highlights how deeply connected your physical and brain health are.

Taking care of your physical health — metabolism, liver, cardiovascular, digestive, and immune systems — directly impacts how your brain functions and feels. Brain health is not just about cognitive challenges or mood management; it's about taking a comprehensive approach that addresses your whole body.

This chapter considers a common health issue plaguing modern humans: Metabolic syndrome, a group of conditions that together raise your risk of cardiovascular disease, stroke, diabetes, and trigger brain health dysfunction and disease.

Characterizing Metabolic Syndrome

Take a moment to understand what metabolism means. You may hear this word a lot, especially when talking about health and well-being.

Understanding the basics of metabolism

Metabolism is the set of chemical reactions in your body that turn the food you eat into energy.

When you eat, your digestive system breaks down the food into basic components such as glucose (sugar), amino acids (from proteins), and fatty acids (from fats). These molecules enter your bloodstream and travel to your cells, where they undergo a series of chemical reactions to fuel essential cellular functions.

The key processes include the following:

>> **Catabolism:** The process where food is broken down into smaller molecules, like carbohydrates into glucose, to produce energy (ATP).

>> **Anabolism:** The process of using molecules from catabolism to build and repair tissues, or synthesize hormones like serotonin from amino acids.

>> **Energy storage:** Excess energy is stored as glycogen in the liver and muscles, or as fat in adipose tissue.

Hormones such as insulin and glucagon play crucial roles in regulating your metabolism, ensuring that your body maintains a balance between energy intake, storage, and use.

REMEMBER

When your metabolism is humming along as it should, it maintains balance in your body and you experience health and well-being. But when the balance is disrupted, you can develop diseases associated with metabolic dysfunction. Often, but not always, metabolism is off balance by things such as poor diet or sedentary living. Some metabolic problems are also genetic.

Defining poor metabolic health

Poor metabolic health occurs when your body's processes become imbalanced, often due to poor diet, lack of exercise, or stress. This imbalance can lead to metabolic syndrome, which raises the risk of heart disease, stroke, and type 2 diabetes. If you have risk factors, your doctor may run tests, check your waist circumference, weight, blood pressure, and possibly refer you for cardiac testing.

Metabolic syndrome is diagnosed when you have at least three of the following conditions:

» **High blood pressure:** 130/85 mmHg or higher

» **High fasting blood sugar:** 100 mg/dL or higher

» **Low HDL cholesterol levels:** Less than 40 mg/dL for men and less than 50 mg/dL for women

» **High triglyceride levels:** 150 mg/dL or higher

» **Abdominal obesity:** A waist circumference of 40 inches or more for men and 35 inches or more for women (although this measurement varies in different parts of the world). Sometimes BMI of over 30 is used here.

All of these problems are interconnected. It's hard to tell which comes first, but many experts believe obesity might trigger metabolic syndrome. Losing weight and staying active help lower triglycerides, improve cholesterol, reduce blood pressure, and improve insulin sensitivity.

High blood pressure

A healthy blood pressure for most people is less than 120/80 mmHg. If your blood pressure is continuously over 130/85 mmHg, you may have high blood pressure or hypertension, one of the indicators of metabolic syndrome.

High blood pressure is a condition in which the force of your blood against the walls of your arteries is consistently too high. Having high blood pressure can damage your arteries and blood vessels reducing blood flow to your brain and other vital organs. Chronic high blood pressure can lead to the formation of stroke, aneurysms, heart failure, and kidney damage.

According to the World Health Organization (WHO), over 1.13 billion people world-wide have high blood pressure, and most of those people are not being treated or taking steps to manage it. Treating high blood pressure includes lifestyle changes such as a healthy diet, regular physical activity, maintaining a healthy weight, cutting your alcohol intake, and avoiding smoking.

High blood sugar

High blood sugar, or *hyperglycemia*, occurs when there's too much glucose in your blood, which can lead to diabetes and increase your risk for heart disease, kidney disease, nerve damage, and dementia. *Insulin*, a hormone from the pancreas, regulates blood sugar, but when your body becomes resistant to it, blood sugar levels rise.

Your blood sugar is usually tested after you've not eaten or fasted for eight to 12 hours. Your blood sugar should be between 70 and 99 mg/dL. If fasting blood sugar level is between 100 and 125 mg/dL you have pre-diabetes. If your blood sugar level is 126 mg/dL or over, you can be suffering from diabetes.

Chronic high blood sugar can damage blood vessels and nerves, leading to complications that affect various parts of your body, including your brain. Over time, this can impair cognitive functions and increase the risk of dementia. Research indicates that people with diabetes are at a higher risk of developing Alzheimer's disease.

Managing blood sugar involves a balanced diet, regular exercise, healthy weight, and medication if needed. A diet rich in vegetables, whole grains, and lean proteins while low in processed foods and sugars is recommended by the Australian Diabetes Society.

Abnormal cholesterol levels

Cholesterol is a waxy molecule found throughout the body. It isn't "bad" per se, unless you get too much of it. Cholesterol originates from two sources: Your liver (which synthesizes all of the cholesterol you need) and your diet (from meat, poultry, and dairy). Your body requires cholesterol to build cells and synthesize vitamins and hormones.

Cholesterol is carried around your body by tiny particles made of lipids and proteins. The two types of lipoproteins are:

>> **Low-density lipoprotein (LDL),** sometimes called "bad" cholesterol

>> **High-density lipoprotein (HDL),** sometimes called "good" cholesterol

If you have high levels of bad cholesterol (LDL) or low levels of good cholesterol (high-density lipoprotein or HDL) your risk of various diseases increases. High LDL cholesterol is partly responsible for the buildup of plaque buildup in your arteries known as atherosclerosis. The plaques narrow your blood vessels and reduce blood flow to your brain and other organs.

Maintaining healthy cholesterol levels involves changing your diet (see Chapter 12), regular exercise (see Chapter 13), avoiding smoking, and taking medication if needed. The National Health and Medical Research Council (NHMRC) of Australia recommends a diet low in saturated fats and high in fruits, vegetables, and whole grains to manage cholesterol levels.

High triglyceride levels

Triglycerides are another type of fat circulating in your blood. They're made by your liver and also come from the food you eat, especially fats (for example, butter, oils, and animal fats). Unused calories are stored as triglycerides in your fat cells. Drinking too much alcohol also contributes to high triglyceride levels.

A healthy level in your blood is below 150 mg/dL for adults or under 90 mg/dL for children and teens.

Rather similarly to high LDLs, high triglycerides may contribute to arteriosclerosis, which increases your risk of stroke, heart attack, and heart disease. Extremely high triglycerides (over 500 mg/dL) can also cause acute inflammation of the pancreas (pancreatitis).

Abdominal obesity

TIP

I get that it is not fashionable to discuss body weight or waist circumference, and over the years, plenty of good work has been done to reduce the kind of fat shaming those of us who came of age in the 1990s accepted as normal. But obesity is not just a cosmetic concern; it's a health problem that increases your risk of other diseases and health problems, such as heart disease, diabetes, high blood pressure, and certain cancers.

Obesity is defined by a body mass index (BMI) of 30 or higher. Although some people prefer to use waist circumference measurements and a tape measure around your waist should show less than 40 inches for men and 35 inches for women. Waist circumference is less accurate for some people (pregnancy being the obvious situation!) and for some populations of people including Aboriginal and Torres Strait Islander peoples in Australia, South Asians, Chinese, and Japanese people.

Risk factors for metabolic syndrome

Multiple factors contribute to metabolic syndrome, and these factors influence one another. Some of these factors are within your control, such as how much exercise you get and what you eat. You have no say over other factors, such your genetic makeup and chronological age.

Uncontrollable risk factors
for metabolic syndrome

Some risk factors for metabolic syndrome are, sadly, beyond your control:

>> **Age:** Your risk increases as you get older.

>> **Socio-economic status:** Low income can lead to poor diet, inactivity, and inadequate sleep.

>> **Family history:** A family history of diabetes or metabolic syndrome increases your risk.

>> **Hormonal conditions:** Polycystic ovary syndrome, immune disorders, or maternal obesity during pregnancy raise your risk.

>> **Sleep issues:** Chronic sleep problems, including sleep apnea and circadian rhythm disorders, can elevate your risk.

>> **Older women are at higher risk:** Older women, especially after menopause, are at higher risk due to hormonal changes.

>> **Some medicines:** Medications for allergies, mental health conditions, HIV, and other illnesses can increase the risk.

Controllable risk factors for metabolic syndrome

Your lifestyle choices play a significant role in your risk of developing metabolic syndrome. Here are some key lifestyle habits that you may have a little more control over than your age, sex, or family history:

>> **Physical inactivity:** Lack of regular exercise increases your risk.

>> **Unhealthy diet:** A diet high in unhealthy foods and large portions contributes to metabolic syndrome.

>> **Poor sleep:** Disrupted sleep affects how your body processes nutrients.

>> **Smoking and alcohol:** Smoking and heavy drinking elevate your risk.

>> **Shift work:** Irregular work hours, especially shift work, can increase your risk.

Linking Metabolic Syndrome to Brain Health

Remember the beginning of this chapter where your brain and body have a conversation about how the health of the body was "messing with mood and memory"? This is not just a light-hearted chit-chat, it's a serious discussion.

Metabolic syndrome increases risk for poor brain health

Being physically unhealthy or living with metabolic syndrome increases your risk of mental illness, faster aging, and dementia.

>> **Mental health:** Metabolic syndrome is linked to depression and anxiety due to inflammation and insulin resistance.

>> **Faster aging:** Poor metabolic health speeds up aging, increasing the risk of cognitive decline.

>> **Dementia:** Metabolic syndrome raises the risk of dementia by damaging blood vessels and neurons.

Poor physical health and poor brain health go together

Chronic diseases such as heart disease, obesity, and diabetes are more common in people who have mental illness. But it's not just metabolic syndrome that is the problem.

A sobering 2023 study from the University of Melbourne involving over 100,000 participants, compared the health of people with serious mental illnesses such as depression, bipolar disorder, and schizophrenia with mentally healthy people. They devised a "body health score" to rate the health of seven different systems of the body (lungs, musculoskeletal, kidney, metabolic, liver, cardiovascular, and immune) and brain health.

People with poor mental health had significantly lower body health scores compared to mentally well people, and their metabolic, liver, and immune systems were particularly unhealthy. Notably, people with schizophrenia showed the poorest brain health, while overall, body health was poorer than brain health for all neuropsychiatric conditions studied.

The researchers put forward a few likely scenarios linking body health, brain health, and mental health, including the following:

>> **Lack of healthcare access:** People with mental illness often miss regular checkups and preventive screenings.

>> **Medications:** Some mental health medications can cause issues like diabetes and obesity.

>> **Chronic stress:** Long-term stress from mental illness can disrupt hormones and harm physical health.

>> **Lifestyle factors:** Unhealthy behaviors like smoking and lack of exercise worsen physical health.

>> **Immune system dysfunction:** Mental health disorders are linked to immune system problems, which can be both a cause and effect.

>> **Faster aging:** Poor physical health can make the body age faster, leading to age-related diseases earlier in life.

Dr. Tian, one of the researchers summed the findings up by saying, "It is important to use a systems and holistic approach to evaluate the health and function of multiple brain and body systems using a variety of organ-specific markers in common mental disorders."

Implementing Preventative Strategies

More than half of all Australians and Americans have at least one of the metabolic syndrome contributors.

Lifestyle changes are extremely important in the management of the metabolic syndrome, but sometimes medication is necessary. Some people need to take tablets to control to keep their blood pressure and cholesterol within the recommended limits. For many people, medications may be the most important step to reduce your risk of heart attack, diabetes, and stroke. Your family doctor is all too familiar with these medications and the risks and benefits.

Getting professional help

Finding a family doctor is a great step toward maintaining your health, especially for men who may be less likely to seek care. Ask friends or family for recommendations, or check with your local health department or insurance company for a list of doctors.

REMEMBER

Remember, a family doctor is not just for when you're unwell, they're essential for preventing health issues before they start.

Making healthy lifestyle changes

TIP

Incorporate as many positive lifestyle changes as you can — eating a healthy diet, exercising regularly, and losing weight can dramatically reduce your risk of diseases associated with metabolic syndrome, such as diabetes and heart disease.

>> **Change your diet.** Focus on whole grains, vegetables, and fruit, and reduce portions and foods high in fat or sugar. Limit alcohol to less than two drinks a day.

>> **Move more.** Aim for 30 minutes of activity at least five days a week, and break up sitting time with short walks.

>> **Lose your belly fat.** Improve eating habits and increase physical activity to reduce excess body fat.

>> **Quit smoking and alcohol.** Both habits increase your risk of serious diseases, and quitting brings many health benefits.

>> **Sleep.** Get 7 to 8 hours of quality sleep each night to support weight control and metabolic health.

>> **Manage stress.** Practice mindfulness, meditation, or deep breathing to reduce stress and improve overall well-being.

REMEMBER

Changing your lifestyle isn't easy, but it's worth it. Small, gradual changes can lead to significant health improvements. Remember, every healthy choice you make is a step towards better brain health.

Chapter **20**

Avoiding Hearing Loss

O kay, brace yourself for a surprising twist in your brain health journey. Caring for your *hearing* can help keep your brain sharp and ward off dementia. Yes, you heard that right (sorry for the bad joke).

Hearing loss is a global issue. In countries with accessible healthcare, like Australia, about one in six people suffer from hearing loss, but most receive treatment. While many gradually lose hearing with age, some are born profoundly deaf or become deaf early in life.

The WHO predicts that by 2050, nearly 2.5 billion people will experience some degree of hearing loss, including many children. For those with disabling hearing loss (over 35 dB in the better ear), nearly 80% live in low- and middle-income countries without proper treatment.

Hearing loss can occur at birth, due to health problems, or from aging, but those in noisy jobs — like construction, music, farming, and the military — face the highest risk.

In this final chapter of this part of the book, you take a quick look at how hearing loss is linked to an increased dementia risk. It may seem like a random addition to the usual suspects of heart health, diet, and exercise, but trust me, the statistics mean this is a brief detour worth taking.

How Hearing Loss Can Lead to Poor Brain Health

Many people are surprised to learn that hearing loss is linked to an increased risk of dementia.

REMEMBER

All Alzheimer's disease and dementia-prevention organizations and government campaigns now encourage the use of hearing aids for hearing loss and recommend protecting your ears from excessive noise exposure.

Surveying the statistics of hearing loss and dementia

WARNING

The 2024 report of the Lancet Commission on dementia prevention, intervention, and care found that hearing loss was *the strongest risk factor* for dementia, accounting for 7 per cent of cases globally.

This conclusion was drawn from a meta-analysis of studies involving people who initially had normal cognitive function but experienced hearing loss at a level of 25 decibels (dB). This level is the threshold defined by the World Health Organization (WHO) for hearing loss. Some real-world examples of this level of hearing loss include:

» Struggling to hear soft sounds such as whispering, rustling leaves, or distant birds chirping

» Finding it hard to catch all the words in a low-volume conversation or have trouble hearing a clock ticking or water dripping

» Difficulty understanding speech in noisy environments, such as a restaurant or a busy street, where background noise can mask softer sounds

TECHNICAL STUFF

The Lancet Commission found that older people with untreated hearing loss were nearly twice as likely to develop dementia over the next nine to 17 years. Because they followed people for such a long time, it was unlikely that the dementia caused the hearing loss. Backing this up, another detailed analysis found that for every 10 dB drop in hearing, the risk of dementia increased by 30 percent. Finally, a large study of over 6,400 Americans, with an average age of 59, showed that even mild hearing loss (less than 25 dB) was linked to lower thinking and memory scores.

Linking hearing loss to dementia

Researchers suspect several plausible mechanisms may link hearing loss to dementia. These mechanisms include the social cost of communication loss, cognitive changes, brain pathology, and a potential shared pathology with dementia.

Social isolation

Hearing loss doesn't just mean your dad needs to turn up the TV volume, your neighbor is always asking people to speak up, or you avoid parties because you can't hear anything. Hearing loss also means you may miss out on conversations at family gatherings, struggle with telephone calls, and feel isolated in social settings.

Hearing loss can lead to social isolation, a known risk factor for dementia. When you struggle to hear, you may withdraw from social interactions, leading to loneliness and depression, which further increase your risk of dementia.

Cognitive change

When you have hearing loss, your brain must work harder to process sounds. This shift in attention can take away cognitive resources needed for other functions such as memory and thinking. All this additional effort can lead to cognitive overload and fatigue and, some scientists suspect, structural changes in your brain, further impacting your cognitive abilities.

The combination of cognitive strain from trying to hear people and the knock-on effect of reduced social engagement creates yet another vicious circle. The more isolated you become, the greater the strain on your brain, which can contribute to cognitive decline and increase your risk of dementia.

Brain structure change

Hearing loss potentially leads to alternations in brain structure and, in one sense, speeds up the aging process. Networks within your brain that are involved in processing sound become less active, which may affect other cognitive functioning over time.

Cognitive reserve, a concept discussed in Chapter 16, refers to your brain's ability to compensate for age-related degeneration. Hearing loss may potentially reduce this reserve, making your brain more vulnerable to dementia.

Shared pathology

Another intriguing possibility is that hearing loss and dementia may share common underlying pathologies, such as vascular issues or neurodegeneration. Although it very much depends on your type of hearing loss (read on in this chapter to discover more), essentially, the same biological processes that cause damage to the auditory system may also harm brain areas responsible for cognitive functions, suggesting that the processes leading to hearing loss may also contribute to cognitive decline.

This upside of the shared pathology theory is that interventions targeting these underlying issues could potentially benefit both hearing and cognitive health.

Recognizing That You May Have Hearing Loss

Hearing loss makes it difficult or impossible to hear speech and other sounds. It ranges from mild to profound and can be temporary or permanent.

TIP

Deafness is the complete loss of your hearing. If you have partial hearing loss, you are known as being "hard of hearing."

Symptoms of hearing loss

Some people don't notice the first signs of hearing loss because they happen slowly. Some of the common symptoms are:

>> Trouble hearing in noisy places

>> Difficulty hearing on the phone or if people aren't facing you

>> Asking people to repeat themselves often

>> Hearing sounds as muffled

>> Needing the TV louder

>> Missing phone or doorbell rings

>> Buzzing or ringing in the ears

>> Avoiding social situations due to hearing difficulties

WARNING

If you experience sudden hearing loss — overnight or in less than three days — you should get medical advice ASAP. There can be plenty of reasons for this, such as an infection or medications, or something more serious such as a stroke or head injury. You have a better chance of getting better if you get help quickly.

TIP

If you're worried about your hearing (or any aspect of your brain health), visit your family doctor. You can find out what kind of hearing loss you have and how bad it is with a hearing test. And if you're unsure whether you have a problem, plenty of free and easy online hearing tests exist. However, a hearing test by an audiologist is the only test that can tell you how well you hear.

Types of hearing loss

Depending on which part of your hearing pathway is affected, there are different types of hearing loss:

>> **Auditory processing disorders:** These happen when your brain has trouble handling sound. It's hard to understand words or figure out where sounds are coming from.

>> **Conductive hearing loss:** That's when something is wrong with your outer or middle ear, and sound can't get to your inner ear. It can be caused by ear wax, an ear infection, or a torn eardrum, or if you have otosclerosis, bones in your middle ear grow in a way that isn't normal. Children are more likely to have treatable conductive hearing loss.

>> **Sensorineural hearing loss:** This disorder is when something is wrong with your auditory nerve or cochlea, the hearing organ in your inner ear. It can be caused by getting older (also called presbycusis), noise-induced hearing loss, infections, Meniere's disease, and some drugs and medicines. A lot of the time, sensorineural hearing loss is permanent.

>> **Presbycusis:** This is a type of sensorineural hearing loss where your hearing gradually deteriorates as you age. It affects about three to four in every ten people over age 65. It's caused by a loss of hair cells in your cochlea, which transduce sound vibrations from your middle ear and sends them as signals through your auditory nerve to your brain. If you've been exposed to excess loud noise, you can experience presbycusis at a younger age.

>> **Mixed hearing loss:** A combination of conductive and sensorineural hearing loss.

Taking Charge of Your Hearing

Because most hearing loss is permanent, preventing it before it begins is critical. If you already have hearing damage, you should take steps to prevent it from worsening

Prevention is better than cure

Restricting your exposure to loud noises is the most effective strategy to safeguard your hearing. This includes events such as loud concerts or building sites (don't avoid Taylor Swift concerts, but perhaps consider earplugs if you're lucky enough to go more than once) and throughout your life. Even an overly loud event or activity can harm your hearing. If you've ever experienced ringing in your ears, ears that feel "full" or "blocked", or sounds that appear fainter afterwards, your hearing has probably been slightly damaged.

To protect your hearing:

>> Keep your music, TV, and radio turned down; you should easily be able to hear someone chatting one meter away.

>> If you're using headphones or earphones, keep the volume low. It should not be audible to someone standing next to you.

>> Protect your ears in noisy environments and during loud activities such as lawn mowing.

>> Take breaks from loud surroundings if possible.

>> If possible, utilize headphones or earphones that block out ambient sounds.

>> Wear earplugs in clubs, live music events, and other loud environments. Take regular breaks and stand further back from the speakers.

>> Follow the rules at work. Many workplaces have strict occupational health and safety rules regarding noise levels.

>> Childhood immunizations are also critical in preventing viral infections that previously caused deafness in children. Before widespread vaccinations, mumps was a leading cause of hearing loss in kids.

Getting help for hearing loss

Can't hear? Don't wait to get treatment! This statement can sum up all the best hearing advice.

Taking steps if you're worried about your hearing

Feeling concerned is a sign to act. Here are situations you should be aware of:

» You may have hearing loss if you notice signs such as turning up the TV volume, asking people to repeat themselves, struggling to hear in noisy places, or ringing in your ears. Feeling concerned is a sign to act.

» Schedule a hearing test with an audiologist. No referral is needed in many parts of the world, but you may need to check with your local doctor for advice.

» If you experience sudden hearing loss, go to your local emergency department.

» Suppose it's not yourself but a child, who shows signs such as delayed speech, unclear speech, not reacting to loud noises, or struggling at school. Don't delay consulting a health professional.

» If a loved one is resistant to getting help, encourage them gently by explaining the benefits of early diagnosis and treatment for their overall quality of life.

Visiting an audiologist

When you visit an audiology clinic, the audiologist starts by performing a hearing test called pure tone audiometry. This test checks how well you can hear different sounds. You wear headphones and listen to various tones to see how well sound travels through your ear canal and middle ear. Then, the audiologist may use a small vibrating device behind your ear to test how well sounds are transmitted through the bone to your inner ear.

Another test that may be done is tympanometry, which checks the pressure in your middle ear and how your eardrum moves. This helps to identify any issues that may be affecting your hearing. After all the tests, the audiologist reviews the results with you, explaining what they find and discussing possible treatments to improve your hearing.

The situation is slightly different for testing hearing in babies and young children. Your child's audiologist chooses from a range of tests and picks those that are best for your child's age.

Exploring treatment options

If you're diagnosed with hearing loss, your treatment options depend on various factors, including the type and severity of your hearing loss, overall health, and personal preferences. All of this should be discussed with your healthcare provider. Audiologists and ear, nose, and throat (ENT) specialists work closely with you to determine the best course of action, considering both the technological options and your lifestyle needs.

The most common therapeutic options (depending on the cause of your hearing loss) include:

>> Hearing Aids

>> Ear wax removal

>> Medication (antibiotics for infections, antihistamines for allergies)

>> Cochlear Implants

>> Bone-anchored hearing systems

Hearing aids

If you're experiencing hearing loss in Australia, a range of advanced hearing aids and treatments are available. These may not be available everywhere, but this list gives you an insight into the range of options. Hearing aids come in various styles to cater to different levels of hearing loss and personal preferences.

>> Behind-the-ear (BTE) hearing aids rest behind your ear and connect to an earmold inside the ear canal, making them suitable for all ages and levels of hearing loss.

>> Receiver-in-Canal (RIC) hearing aids are similar but smaller and less visible, providing natural sound quality.

>> In-the-ear (ITE) aids fit the outer ear and are discreet and easy to handle, which is ideal for mild to severe hearing loss.

>> For even more discretion, In-the-Canal (ITC) and Completely-in-Canal (CIC) aids fit wholly or partly inside the ear canal, making them nearly invisible and perfect for mild to moderate hearing loss.

Implants

If you have severe to profound hearing loss and hearing aids won't benefit you, cochlear implants may be the solution.

Cochlear implants and hearing aids work very differently. Hearing aids boost sounds so that people can hear them. Cochlear implants bypass damaged parts of the ear and stimulate the auditory nerve directly; the brain interprets these signals as sound. Learning or relearning how to hear with a cochlear implant takes time because it's different from everyday hearing.

>> **Bone conduction hearing aids** transmit sound through the bones of your skull, bypassing the outer and middle ear, making them effective if you have conductive hearing loss or single-sided deafness.

>> **Middle ear implants** are surgically placed devices that mechanically stimulate the structures of the middle ear and are suitable if you have sensorineural hearing loss and cannot wear conventional hearing aids.

Surgical treatments

For some cases of hearing loss, auditory brainstem implants are available. These devices bypass the cochlea and auditory nerve entirely, directly stimulating the brainstem, which is especially useful if you have auditory nerve damage.

Listening to Advice on Hearing Loss

Treating hearing loss is crucial for your brain health and should be one of the most essential parts of your dementia-risk reduction plan.

WARNING

Studies show that older adults with hearing problems are more likely to develop dementia *unless they use hearing aids*. The Lancet Commission's research, with thousands of participants over many years, found that those who started using hearing aids experienced less memory decline.

REMEMBER

Hearing aids help you hear better and keep your brain active and engaged, protecting against cognitive decline. So, by addressing hearing loss, you're not just improving your hearing — you're also taking a significant step to safeguard your brain health.

6

The Part of Tens

Examine lifestyle choices that will damage your brain.

Recogize the functions of a healthy, high-performing brain.

Chapter **21**

Ten Ways to Hurt Your Happy, Healthy Brain

As I wrap up this book, I thought we should have a little fun.

It's hard not to get bogged down in serious conversations about depression, dementia, and dysfunction when it comes to health and well-being. So, to lighten the mood, I explore what not to do if you want a happy, healthy high-performing brain.

Here are ten surefire ways to sabotage your brain's health, served with a lashing of my best (worst) jokes.

Get ready to roll your eyes so hard you'll see your own brain.

Never Get Enough Sleep

Want to sabotage your brain? Skimp on your sleep!

Treat your brain like a high-performance engine that never needs a tune-up. Skip the necessary seven to eight hours of sleep and try to mix up your bedtime: Go to bed at 3 a.m. one day and 7 p.m. the next. Sleep in one day and get up early the next. The more irregular your routines, the less likely you'll sleep well.

Then, watch as your brain struggles to consolidate memories and regulate emotions. With any luck, you feel cranky and may even end up with brain fog. Chronic sleep deprivation leads to anxiety, depression, heart disease, diabetes, and dementia. Ask yourself: Who needs a well-rested brain anyway? Not you, you hybrid night owl/morning lark!

If you're a parent, you can make life even more chaotic and tiring. Ignore all the best health advice and let your kids decide when they want to go to bed. And when they do hit the sack, encourage them to scroll through social media on their phones until the wee small hours. They'll be miserable the next day, won't enjoy school, and you'll ensure their brains are in no fit state to learn and grow.

Become a Hermit

Humans are tribe animals, so if you're looking for one of the most effective ways to hurt your brain, avoid meaningful social connections.

By isolating yourself from your community and experiencing solitude and true loneliness, you deprive your brain of the chance to engage in the dynamic and challenging social interactions it craves. You may start to feel sad and even sink into depression, and your long-term brain health prospects will start to dim. Before you know it, you'll be on the path towards dementia.

Instead of catching up with your best friend over coffee, opt to stay home and scroll through social media. You'll miss out on those laughs, shared stories, and the subtle cognitive stimulation that comes from reading facial expressions, tone of voice, and body language. When you avoid community activities, you also miss out on opportunities to build cognitive reserve through learning and adapting to new social environments. Ultimately, you're robbing your brain of the rich, rewarding experiences that keep it sharp and resilient. Go it alone.

Stress Yourself Out

Want to wreak havoc on your brain? Stress out constantly! Seek out those situations or people you know grind your gears. Or spend some time ruminating over a past failure or future catastrophe. Let it consume your thoughts. Rumination is a bit like sitting on a rocking chair — you keep yourself busy but get nowhere. Really lean into the stressful feelings.

Remember that toxic or chronic stress wreaks havoc on your body and brain and can send you into an allostatic downward spiral.

Living in a heightened state of stress keeps your brain on high alert, leaving you exhausted and less capable of handling day-to-day life. Over time, your constant state of stress can lead to anxiety, depression, and even physical health issues such as heart disease.

Pursue less useful ways of building resilience, such as day drinking, eating junk food, or hours of mindless doom-scrolling (combine all three!). And forget about mindfulness and meditation (unless you're a teenager, then try to convince your school to stress you all out by forcing you to complete MBSR training every week). Some of you may even feel worse than before.

So go ahead, embrace the chaos and watch your brain's health spiral downwards.

Eat Junk Food

A diet high in ultra-processed foods and sugar is perfect for creating metabolic disorders and inflammation. Avoid fruits, veggies, whole grains, lean proteins, and healthy fats at all costs. Prioritize the following: Sugary cereals, fast food, sodas, and anything that comes from a factory wrapped in a crinkly package with a long list of unpronounceable ingredients.

If you keep this up, you'll be one step closer to developing depression, metabolic health syndrome, and even dementia.

Forget about the Mediterranean diet. Embrace the junk food lifestyle and watch your cognitive functions decline. Remember, the worse the fuel, the faster your brain deteriorates.

Enjoy that brain fog alongside the hot chips and donuts!

Lay Around Doing Nothing

Physical activity is great for brain health and one of the best tools to slow aging. Regular exercise helps regulate blood sugar, reduce inflammation, and lower stress hormone levels. So, to harm your brain, it's best to lay around and do nothing!

Muscle is like a longevity organ, releasing signaling molecules that promote brain health. So, it's best to let them waste away. Avoid resistance training and multi-component exercises at all costs — they enhance cognitive function and protect against aging.

Skip aerobic activities, strength training, and balance exercises. And never ever consider walking the dog, going for a swim, team sports with other people, or sports that challenge your mind.

Make laziness a regular part of your routine and watch your brain decline. Embrace the couch potato life!

Blast the Music and Ditch the Bike Helmet

Hearing loss is more than an inconvenience; it can lead to social isolation, depression, and increase your risk of dementia. To double your risk of dementia as you age, ensure your hearing loss remains untreated. Never talk to the doctor about getting your hearing tested or getting hearing aids.

Why not crank up the volume on your headphones to the max and enjoy those sweet tunes until your ears ring? Forget about those silly earplugs at concerts — stand right next to the speakers and feel the bass shake your bones. If your ears ring the next day — well done! You've damaged some hair cells in your cochlea.

Let your brain disengage and watch cognitive decline take over.

Brain injuries or concussions from sports, accidents, or falls devastate cognitive function. Ignoring the need to wear protective gear such as helmets while cycling, never buckling your seatbelt, or playing contact sports invites disaster. Climb that ladder to clear the leaves from the gutter. Show the youngsters you're as fit and nimble as you always were.

Why protect your brain when you can just let it get damaged?

Avoid Ever Learning Anything New

Your brain loves a good challenge, so to hurt it, avoid lifelong learning. If you were privileged enough to complete high school and attend college, and you're now gainfully employed in a stimulating job you love, I'm sorry, all that education and intellectual stimulation is providing you protection against brain aging.

However, all is not lost: Skip learning a new language or playing an instrument, forget about Wordle, and for goodness' sake, don't read a book. Another tip is to retire as early as possible. You'll have more time to "lay around doing nothing" (see the previous section).

Avoid building cognitive reserve, a buffer against aging and neurodegenerative diseases. By refusing to challenge your brain — especially after you're retired, you ensure a nice steady decline in cognitive function and increase your dementia risk.

Who needs education or intellectual stimulation anyway?

Drink and Take Illicit Drugs (Daily)

Certain substances are particularly harmful to your brain. To really mess it up, drink daily, get yourself addicted to tobacco like it's the 1970s again, and really lean into those "recreational drugs." Depending on where you live in the world, those drugs may land you in jail, so choose wisely.

Water quality and access? Pfft, who needs clean water when you can live life on the edge? Remember, one in four people worldwide lack access to clean drinking water, and around one million people die every year from unsafe water and poor hygiene. So, if you really want to mess up your health, start by ignoring your water intake. You can even take your dehydrated self to the side of a busy highway and breathe in those traffic fumes.

Live a polluted life. Double your risk of brain damage!

Avoid Joy and Wallow around in Doom and Gloom

Positive emotions such as joy, satisfaction, contentment, or anticipation are great for mental well-being and tangible benefits for brain health. So, if you're aiming for cognitive decline, make sure to shun joy, gratitude, and contentment. And don't ever start a gratitude journal — because who needs daily reminders of positivity?

One way to find activities that bring purpose, passion, and optimism into your life is to ask yourself: "Is it awesome, and does it help?" Tip: Don't ask yourself that question.

To really ensure your mental health goes downhill, avoid activities that bring you joy. Skip spending time in nature, ditch enjoyable silly hobbies, and never, ever laugh with friends.

Neglect your emotional well-being and create a negative feedback loop that drags down your quality of life and brain function. Remember, a miserable mind is an unhealthy mind. So, make sure to avoid anything that makes you smile!

Aim for gloom and doom and watch your brain wilt like an unwatered plant.

Embrace the Couch and Cake Life

Metabolic disorders such as diabetes, obesity, and hypertension are closely linked to brain health issues. To destroy your brain, make sure to ignore a healthy diet by indulging in fast food, sugary snacks, and processed meals packed with preservatives. Avoid regular physical activity and neglect stress management entirely. Skip regular checkups to monitor blood sugar, cholesterol, and blood pressure levels (and if you have a trusted family doctor, don't discuss anything with them — they may refer you for specialized care).

Early intervention and lifestyle changes can prevent or mitigate these disorders' impact on your brain. But who cares? What's good for your heart is also good for your brain, so avoid heart-healthy habits and let both suffer.

Embrace metabolic disorders through unhealthy living.

Chapter **22**

Ten Functions of a High-Performing, Happy, Healthy Brain

Congratulations! You made it to the end of our exploration of the human brain.

The journey to understanding your brain may have seemed daunting at the beginning of this book. After all, to some people neuroscience sounds as overwhelming as rocket surgery! I hope you gained a comprehensive understanding of how your brain and body work together to create your unique experience of being you.

In this final chapter, you'll look at a few feats a happy, healthy, high-performance brain can do: enhanced memory, sharp focus, emotional resilience, creativity, and overall cognitive agility. Embrace these potentials and continue your journey towards optimal brain health.

With this knowledge, you're well-equipped to maintain the health of your brain and those of your loved ones. Keep nurturing your brain, stay curious, and remember that the journey to brain health is a lifelong adventure.

Cognitive Abilities: Your Brain's CEO

Cognitive abilities encompass a range of mental processes, including reasoning, problem-solving, and critical thinking. Your brain's cortex, particularly the frontal and parietal lobes, plays a crucial role in performing these duties.

The Executive Network brings together different regions of your brain to facilitate complex mental tasks. It's like the CEO of your brain, directing attention, planning, and coordinating actions. These advanced executive functioning skills set you apart from other mammals, enabling you to filter distractions, prioritize tasks, set and achieve goals, and control impulses in ways other animals can't.

Imagine yourself tackling a tricky Wordle puzzle. Your brain's cognitive skills kick in, analyzing letter clues, spotting patterns, and systematically working towards a solution. This showcases your brain's executive function, demonstrating how a sharp mind helps you tackle complex tasks, and stay on top of your game (and hopefully beat your friends).

Learning and Memory: Your Brain's Dynamic Workshop

Your brain is less like a library than a writer's workshop within a library, where authors constantly gather to write and rewrite stories. Instead of static books on shelves, imagine your memories as evolving manuscripts, edited each time you recall them.

Consider learning to drive. Initially overwhelming, it's like entering a workshop filled with scattered notes and drafts. As you practice, your brain organizes this information, enabling you to recall and perform driving tasks effortlessly. Your brain is not just a repository of information; it's a dynamic learning machine, predicting what to do next based on past experiences.

Imagine driving a familiar route home. Your brain, with its workshop-like adaptability, anticipates turns and signals, automating the task and freeing up mental resources. This efficiency highlights your brain's remarkable capability to navigate a complex world seamlessly, ensuring you can focus on new challenges and learning opportunities.

Attention and Focus: Your Brain's Spotlight

Attention and focus are like a spotlight that helps your brain concentrate on specific tasks while ignoring distractions. Your prefrontal cortex, located at the front of your brain, directs this spotlight, enabling you to stay on task and complete activities efficiently.

Think of a student studying for an exam. Despite the noise and distractions around them, they can zero in on their textbooks and retain the necessary information. This ability to focus and maintain attention is crucial for academic success and everyday tasks.

Recognition of People: Your Brain's Face Detector

Humans are tribe animals, and our brains are wired to connect with others. Think of your brain as a bustling networking event, where people (neurons) constantly mingle and exchange information. You need these neural systems to support social behaviors for survival and thriving. From understanding social cues (these include what you see hear, and even smell!) to responding appropriately, your brain is hard at work, ensuring you can navigate the social world smoothly.

Your brain has specialized networks that help you perceive, understand, and react to social information. These networks include regions that help you decipher faces, make sense of language, and take a pretty good guess at what someone else is thinking or feeling.

Picture this: You're at a party and spot a couple of friends you haven't seen in ages. You wave enthusiastically, and they wave back with equal excitement. As you chat, you laugh at old memories and new jokes, feeling that warm, fuzzy collective vibe. This is your social brain in action, effortlessly making you feel like part of the tribe. So next time you enjoy a good conversation or share a laugh, thank your social brain for keeping you connected and thriving.

Language Capacity: Your Brain's Translator

Language is one of the most complex functions your brain performs. The left hemisphere, particularly Broca's and Wernicke's areas, is involved in producing and understanding speech. These regions process sounds, form words, and create meaningful sentences.

Consider having a conversation with a friend. Your brain seamlessly translates thoughts into words, enabling smooth communication. This intricate process involves multiple brain regions working in harmony, showcasing the brain's incredible capacity for language.

Navigational Skills: Your Brain's GPS

Your brain's hippocampus acts like an internal GPS, helping you navigate your environment — it's not just for making new memories! This spatial memory system enables you to remember routes, landmarks, and directions, meaning you find your way around the world. But your internal GPS does more than just guide you; it thrives on movement.

And movement is more than just exercise; it's essential for keeping your brain healthy. Our brains evolved to help us move, hunt, and gather. When you're active, your brain stays alert and ready for action. But when you sit still for too long, your brain goes into energy-saving mode. Staying active keeps your brain sharp, boosting your ability to plan, remember, and navigate.

Think of finding your way around a new city on holidays. Your brain creates a mental map, helping you remember key locations and find your way back to your hotel room. This navigational ability showcases your brain at peak performance, efficiently processing and storing information to help you explore and thrive in new environments.

Emotional Regulation: Your Brain's Mood Manager

Emotional regulation is your brain's ability to appropriately manage and respond to feelings. The theory of "constructed emotions" explains how your brain creates emotions from a mix of biology, context, and experience. Your brain uses interoception (awareness of internal body states), sensory input, and past experiences to shape your feelings. It's like your brain is an artist, using a palette of sensations, surroundings, and learned vocabulary to paint your feelings. When you're physiologically healthy, you manage emotions effectively, making them a vibrant part of your life rather than a disruptive force.

Consider facing a stressful situation at work. Instead of reacting impulsively, your brain helps you stay calm and think rationally. This emotional regulation is crucial for healthy relationships and mental health. Emotions add color to our lives, making experiences richer and more meaningful.

Stress Management: Your Brain's Chill Pill

Life is full of challenges, and your body's stress response systems help you deal with all sorts of threats, challenges, and opportunities. Stress is an essential neural and physiological response crucial for your survival. It's more than just about being scared or responding with "fight or flight"; it's an orchestrated neuro-symphony that prepares you to adapt and respond effectively. When these systems perform well, your body can return to a healthy baseline, maintaining balance and well-being.

Imagine you're about to compete in a big sporting event — like throwing a javelin at the Olympics! Instead of freezing or running away, your brain orchestrates a symphony of responses: your heart rate increases slightly, adrenaline kicks in, and your mind sharpens. You feel alert and ready, your muscles are primed for action, and your focus is honed on your grip and run-up. After the throw, your body naturally returns to a calm state. This well-regulated stress response enables you to perform at your best and recover quickly. You're adaptable and resilient!

Creative Potential: Your Brain's Artist

Your brain's conscious grey and white matter, which somehow came to life nestled between two eternities of the universe, has enabled humans just like you to achieve incredible feats. Human brains landed on the moon with Apollo 1, decoded the human genome in 2003, painted impressionist water lilies, and built the Sydney Opera House. Human imagination and creativity have continually pushed the boundaries of what's possible and beautiful.

Now, think about kids playing. Their imagination can run wild, turning a cardboard box into a spaceship (or trap their brother inside, duct-taping it shut, and rolling him down a hill), or craft little wooden surfboards. They invent complex rules for handball games or draw pictures that describe other people's feelings. Their little brains solve problems and make sense of the world through creative play. It's the same brain power that helps us all do amazing things. By encouraging and praising this creativity, you'll lay the groundwork for future inventions and discoveries.

Sense of Self: Your Brain's Dream Machine

Your brain's *Default Mode Network* (DMN) is like your personal life planner, responsible for your sense of self, your autobiographical life story, and ability to imagine the future and set goals. When you're not focused on the outside world, your DMN kicks in, engaging in self-referential thoughts and emotions, and thinking about the past or imagining the future. It's the network that helps you reflect on who you are, how you fit into the world, and what you want to achieve.

Imagine the DMN as your brain's storyteller and visionary. It helps you turn your life experiences into a coherent narrative, making sense of who you are today. At the same time, it's busy dreaming up future scenarios, setting goals, and figuring out how to achieve them.

Think about writing a book (I do not need to simply imagine this task!). When you're not writing, your DMN is hard at work, drawing from your wealth of experiences, knowledge, and emotions to craft ideas for each chapter. It's not just about putting words on paper; it's about connecting your personal narrative with the story you want to tell. As you imagine the impact your book will have on readers and set goals for your writing journey, your DMN integrates past successes and future aspirations. (And before you know it, you'll be writing the very last sentence in the book.)

Index

E

early childhood education, 89–92
eating disorders, 110
echolalia, 46
ecstasy, 307–309
education
  cognitive reserve and, 265–266
  early childhood, 89–92
  exercise and, 211
  sleep and, 237
  socioeconomic status and, 185
educational neuroscience specialists, 33
Educational Psychology Review, 211
EEG (electroencephalography), 34, 253
emotional contagion, 252
Emotional Network, 29
emotional regulation, 342–343
emotionally responsive relationships, 87–88
emotions, 10, 130
empathy, 88, 250, 251–252
empathy network, 249
employment, 154, 237, 266
encephalitis, 172
endocannabinoids, 304
Energy Conservation Theory, 224
enteric nervous system (ENS), 15, 201
environment
  air quality, 180
  autumn brain, 183
  environmental toxins, 181
  overview, 179
  seasonal affective disorder, 182
  socioeconomic status, 184–185
  time zone changes, 182
  urban versus rural living, 183–184
  water quality and access, 181
environmental enrichment, 265
environmental nudging, 219–220
epidemiology, 33, 35
epilepsy, 57, 197–198
epinephrine, 21
Escapers, 124
estrogen, 103, 147–148, 154–155

eustress, 93, 279
evidence-based medicine, 36
executive functions, 10, 89–90
Executive Network, 28
exercise
  biological impact of, 214–216
  childhood brain health and, 211
  cognitive decline, battling with, 213–214
  dementia, battling with, 213–214
  environmental nudging, 219–220
  government guidelines, 209–210
  habit formation, 216–219
  intensities, 209
  mood disorders, treating with, 212–213
  overview, 11, 207
  sedentary living and brain health, 208–209, 336
  social support networks, 220
  through evolutionary lens, 208
  types of, 209
experience of stress, 278–279
experience-dependent plasticity, 101
experimental studies, 35
externalizing disorders, 151

F

facial recognition, 341
familial Alzheimer's disease (FAD), 64
family doctors, 37
family history, 72
FASD (fetal alcohol spectrum disorder), 173
F.A.S.T test, 61
fat, dietary, 190
fatherhood, 148
fatigue, 237
fawn response, 287, 288
fencing posture, 79
fermented foods, 204
fetal alcohol spectrum disorder (FASD), 173
fetal brain development, 78–79, 104, 173, 291
FFA (fusiform face area), 107
first 1000-day period, 84–86
first-person language, 41
fish oil, 206

M

machine learning, 34

macronutrients, 190

magnetic resonance imaging (MRI), 34

Maki, Pauline, 162, 163

mama bear responses, 256–257

Man Who Mistook His Wife for a Hat, The (Sacks), 31–32

marijuana, 113–114, 303–306

markers of brain aging, 127–131

Marlin, Bianca Jones, 256

maternal health, 84–85

MBSR (Mindfulness-Based Stress Reduction), 294–295

McEwan, Bruce, 289

MCI (mild cognitive impairment), 135–137, 214

MDMA, 307–309

meaningful work, 11

meditation, 294–295

Mediterranean diet, 193–197

medulla oblongata, 18

melatonin, 115, 182, 233–234

memory, 137, 228–229, 264–265, 340

memory consolidation, 228

Memory Processing Theory, 224

men

  aging and, 151–152

  bio-psycho-social model, 144–145

  heart health, impact on, 153

  hormonal influences in, 152–153

  male sex hormones, 148–150

  mental health disorders in, 153–154

  mood disorders in, 151

  neurodevelopmental disorders in, 150

  neurological disorders in, 153

  occupational hazards and, 154

  overview, 142–143

  sex differences and sexual dimorphism, 143–144

  suicide among, 154

meningitis, 172

menopause

  brain changes during, 160–161

  brain fog in, 162

  common symptoms of, 160

  hormone therapy for, 163–164

  hormone-sensitive subgroups, 164–165

  hot flashes and night sweats in, 161

  mental health and, 163

  overview, 160

  personal differences in, 162–163

menstrual cycle, 154–155

mental challenges and brain games, 268–269

mental health disorders. *See also* anxiety; depression; schizophrenia

  in adolescence, 110–113

  after TBI, 175

  bipolar disorder, 51–52

  ketogenic diet and, 198

  in men, 153–154

  in menopause, 163

  overview, 47

  physical health and, 194

  poor health and, 317–318

  PTSD, 53–55, 291–292

mental health screening, 38

mental skills, differentiating, 131–134

mentalizing network, 249

mesencephalon, 18

metabolic syndrome

  abdominal obesity in, 313, 315

  abnormal cholesterol levels in, 313, 314

  basics of metabolism, 312

  brain health, impact on, 317–318

  chronic stress and, 292

  diagnosis of, 313

  high blood pressure in, 313

  high blood sugar in, 313–314

  high triglyceride levels in, 313, 315

  overview, 200, 311

  preventing, 318–319, 338

  risk factors for, 316–317

  sleep and, 238–239

metabolism, 199–200, 312

microbiome in gut, 202–204

micro-dosing, 308

microglia, 26, 27

micronutrients, 190

midbrain, 18

migraine, 55–56

neuropsychological assessment, 35, 37

neuroscience
  brain health assessments, 36–40
  defined, 32
  related disciplines and professions, 32–33
  research tools and techniques, 33–35
  study design and levels of evidence, 35–36

neurosurgeons, 32

neuro-symphony of stress
  dual stress response system, 283–285
  overview, 282–283
  stress hormones, 286–289

neurotransmitters, 24, 25

New England Centenarian Study (NECS), 124, 125

newborn reflexes, 79–80

NfL (neurofilament light chain), 131

night sweats, 161

non-rapid eye movement (NREM) sleep, 225–227, 228

noradrenaline, 21, 25, 286, 287

norepinephrine, 21

nucleus accumbens (NAcc), 18, 107, 109

nutrition
  antioxidants, 191
  childhood brain development and, 85–86
  coffee, 205, 230–231
  dementia and, 196–197
  fish oil, 206
  food as fuel, 190
  food as signal, 191
  gut-brain axis, 200–204
  intermittent fasting, 206
  junk food, harm caused by, 335
  ketogenic diet, 197–198
  macronutrients and micronutrients, 190
  Mediterranean diet, 193–194
  metabolism, 199–200
  mood disorders and, 195–196
  neuronal health and, 199–200
  overview, 11, 189
  physical health, importance in mental health, 194–195
  red wine, effects of, 205, 302–303
  research challenges, 191–192

societal factors, 192
sugar cravings, 206

O

obesity, 200
observational studies, 35
obstructive sleep apnea (OSA), 238
occipital lobes, 16
occupational complexity, 266
occupational hazards, 154
occupational assessments, 38
oligodendrocytes, 26, 27
open head injury, 168
orbitofrontal cortex (OFC), 106
organization phase, 104
OSA (obstructive sleep apnea), 238
out-of-home childcare, 91–92
ovarian hormones, 147
oxytocin, 255–258

P

PACES (protective factors for adverse childhood experiences), 95–96
parasympathetic nervous system (PSNS), 15, 21, 201, 284, 285
parentese, 88
parents. See childhood brain development
parietal lobes, 16
Parkinson's disease (PD), 64–65, 152, 153
PASA model (Posterior-Anterior Shift in Aging), 130
patient history, 37
peer approval, 109
perception stage, 249
perimenopause, 160
peripheral nervous system (PNS), 14–15, 20
personality traits and, 270–271
Pes, Gianni, 124
PET (positron emission tomography), 34
PFC (prefrontal cortex), 43, 48, 99, 106
physical activity. See exercise
physical examinations, 37
physical health, importance in mental health, 194–195

reductionist view, 28

rehabilitation professionals, 33

relationships, social. *See* social relationships

Relationships in Time and the Life Course: The Significance of Linked Lives, 244

relative risk (RR), 70–71

REM (rapid eye movement) sleep, 225–227, 228, 229

reminiscence bump, 101

research tools and techniques, 33–35

resilience
  building, 292–296
  social relationships and, 95–96

responsive relationships, childhood brain development and, 88

Restorative Theory, 224

reticular formation, 18

retrospective cohort, 36

Reward Sensitivity Model, 110

risk factors
  absolute versus relative risk, 70–71
  genetic, 72
  holistic view of brain health, 73–74
  lifestyle choices and, 73
  overview, 69
  prevalence and incidence, 71–72
  weighing up risks and benefits, 70

risk-taking, in adolescence, 99, 109–110, 116

road safety, 177

roid rage, 149

rooting reflex, 79

RR (relative risk), 70–71

S

Sacks, Oliver, 31–32

SAD (seasonal affective disorder), 182

SAGE (Self-Administered Gerocognitive Exam), 137

Salience Network, 28

schizophrenia
  in adolescents, 111, 114
  cannabis and, 306
  city living as risk for, 183
  ketogenic diet and, 198
  neurobiology of, 53
  overview, 52

symptoms and diagnosis, 52
  treatment options, 53

screening tools, 136

seasonal affective disorder (SAD), 182

second impact syndrome (SIS), 171

second-person neuroscience, 252–253

secure attachments, 245–246

sedentary behavior, 208–209, 336

Self-Administered Gerocognitive Exam (SAGE), 137

self-assessment of brain health, 39–40

self-harm, 111

self-identity, 107–108

sense of self, 108, 344

sensitive periods for brain development, 82–84

sensorineural hearing loss, 325

sensory processing, 9, 19, 20, 130

serotonin, 25, 56

serve and return interactions, 88–89

SES (socioeconomic status), 184–185

Settersten, Richard A., Jr., 244

sex and gender differences
  bio-psycho-social approach to, 144–145
  in brain aging, 151–152
  female sex hormones, 147–148
  male sex hormones, 148–150
  men's brain health, 152–154
  in mood disorders, 151
  in neurodevelopmental disorders, 150
  overview, 142–143
  sex differences and sexual dimorphism, 143–144
  women's brain health
    hormonal contraceptives and, 156
    in menopause, 160–165
    menstrual cycle, 154–155
    overview, 154
    PMS and PMDD, 155
    in pregnancy and motherhood, 156–160

sex hormones
  brain development and, 105
  brain reorganization and, 103–104
  female, 147–148
  general discussion, 102–103
  impact on mood and behavior, 105–106
  male, 148–150, 152–153

About the Author

Dr. Sarah McKay is a neuroscientist and science communicator skilled at making brain science accessible for improving health, well-being, and performance.

An Oxford University graduate, Sarah earned her MSc and DPhil in neuroscience before moving to Australia, where she spent five years doing postdoctoral research on spinal cord injury. After realizing how much people wanted to better understand their brains, she founded the Neuroscience Academy, an online education company for professional development training in applied neuroscience and brain health.

Since hanging up her lab coat, Sarah has been "explaining the brain" on TV, radio, podcasts, and from the stage. Whether on screen, over the airwaves, or in front of an audience, she's committed to making neuroscience simple, engaging, and user-friendly.

She has a special interest in women's brain health and has written two books on the topic: *The Women's Brain Book: The neuroscience of health, hormones, and happiness* and *Baby Brain: The surprising neuroscience of how pregnancy and motherhood sculpt our brains and change our minds (for the better)*.

Sarah lives on Sydney's Northern Beaches with her husband, their two teenage sons (who rarely listen to her brain facts), and one springer spaniel, Albie, who loyally listens to everything. They can often be found surfing, sailing, and swimming in the ocean (sometimes all on the same day!).

Dedication

For my Neuroscience Academy students.

Our conversations over the past decade have taught me what truly matters in brain health. Here's to the neuroscience we've explored together and the questions waiting to be asked.

Author's Acknowledgments

To the scientists whose decades of work gathering, analyzing, and sharing data have made this book possible, your dedication is the foundation of everything we know. It's a privilege to share your research. Any errors in discussing your work are entirely my own.

To my neuroscience students of the past decade: Your questions and conversations have shaped how I communicate complex ideas. I've learned as much from you as you may have learned from me.

To Tim Gallan at Wiley, your diligence and responsiveness have been invaluable. You just get it, and working with you has made this process so much smoother. A special thanks also to Tracy Boggier for asking me to write this book. What a privilege it is to be an author for this iconic brand.

A heartfelt thanks to two key people: Jeanne Ryckmans and Lou Johnson. Without your support and professionalism, I wouldn't have written one, let alone three (!) books.

To my Northern Beaches community, how lucky are we to live in the most glorious corner of Planet Earth? It keeps us happy, healthy, and surrounded by the funniest, most fun people I know.

To our new pup Albie, who reminds us every day that these are the "good old days," giving 110 percent to everything you do and keeping us walking the bush and beaches.

To my family, Geoffrey, Harry, and Jamie, thanks for making sure I never take myself too seriously! And especially to my two boys, you've given me and your Dad real-life courses in parenthood, love, and resilience. Your energy and escapades keep our brains challenged every day.

Publisher's Acknowledgments

Executive Editor: Tracy Boggier
Senior Managing Editor: Kristie Pyles
Development Editor: Tim Gallan
Copy Editor: Jerelind Charles
Technical Editor: Joseph P. Bush, PhD

Production Editor: Saikarthick Kumarasamy
Cover Image: © haerul/Adobe Stock Photos

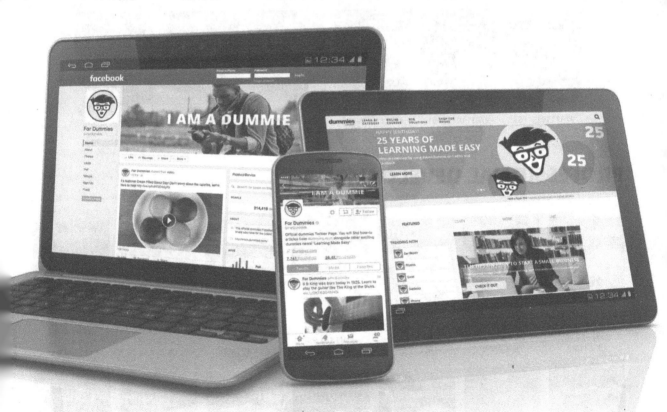
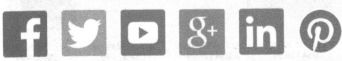

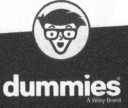

PERSONAL ENRICHMENT

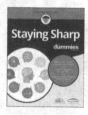
Staying Sharp
9781119187790
USA $26.00
CAN $31.99
UK £19.99

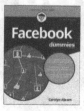
Facebook
9781119179030
USA $21.99
CAN $25.99
UK £16.99

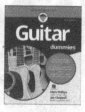
Guitar
9781119293354
USA $24.99
CAN $29.99
UK £17.99

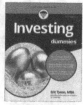
Investing
9781119293347
USA $22.99
CAN $27.99
UK £16.99

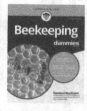
Beekeeping
9781119310068
USA $22.99
CAN $27.99
UK £16.99

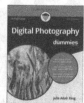
Digital Photography
9781119235606
USA $24.99
CAN $29.99
UK £17.99

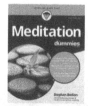
Meditation
9781119251163
USA $24.99
CAN $29.99
UK £17.99

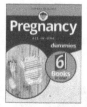
Pregnancy
9781119235491
USA $26.99
CAN $31.99
UK £19.99

Samsung Galaxy S7
9781119279952
USA $24.99
CAN $29.99
UK £17.99

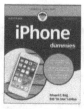
iPhone
9781119283133
USA $24.99
CAN $29.99
UK £17.99

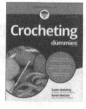
Crocheting
9781119287117
USA $24.99
CAN $29.99
UK £16.99

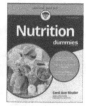
Nutrition
9781119130246
USA $22.99
CAN $27.99
UK £16.99

PROFESSIONAL DEVELOPMENT

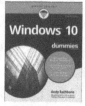
Windows 10
9781119311041
USA $24.99
CAN $29.99
UK £17.99

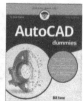
AutoCAD
9781119255796
USA $39.99
CAN $47.99
UK £27.99

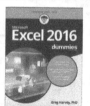
Excel 2016
9781119293439
USA $26.99
CAN $31.99
UK £19.99

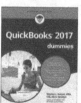
QuickBooks 2017
9781119281467
USA $26.99
CAN $31.99
UK £19.99

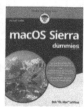
macOS Sierra
9781119280651
USA $29.99
CAN $35.99
UK £21.99

LinkedIn
9781119251132
USA $24.99
CAN $29.99
UK £17.99

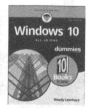
Windows 10
9781119310563
USA $34.00
CAN $41.99
UK £24.99

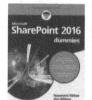
SharePoint 2016
9781119181705
USA $29.99
CAN $35.99
UK £21.99

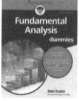
Fundamental Analysis
9781119263593
USA $26.99
CAN $31.99
UK £19.99

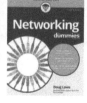
Networking
9781119257769
USA $29.99
CAN $35.99
UK £21.99

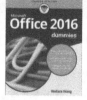
Office 2016
9781119293477
USA $26.99
CAN $31.99
UK £19.99

Office 365
9781119265313
USA $24.99
CAN $29.99
UK £17.99

Salesforce.com
9781119239314
USA $29.99
CAN $35.99
UK £21.99

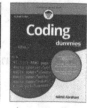
Coding
9781119293323
USA $29.99
CAN $35.99
UK £21.99

dummies.com

dummies
A Wiley Brand